Biomedical Application of 4-Hexylresorcinol

Seong-Gon Kim

Biomedical Application of 4-Hexylresorcinol

Springer

Seong-Gon Kim
Oral and Maxillofacial Surgery
Gangneung–Wonju National University
Gangneung, Kangwon-do, Korea (Republic of)

ISBN 978-981-97-0636-5 ISBN 978-981-97-0637-2 (eBook)
https://doi.org/10.1007/978-981-97-0637-2

This Springer imprint is published by the registered company Springer Nature Singapore Pte Ltd.
The registered company address is: 152 Beach Road, #21-01/04 Gateway East, Singapore 189721, Singapore

Paper in this product is recyclable.

Foreword

Phenolic lipids with a single aromatic ring and non-isoprenoid side chain are widely spread among living organisms and possess plural biological functions. The first mention of phenolic lipids from the plant *Gingko biloba* in the scientific literature goes backs to the early 1930s, and these substances were thought to occur in the certain plant species only. Later, a variety of structures with different side chain length and position at the aromatic ring has been identified in many plant species and microorganisms. Phenolic lipid molecules have hydrophilic benzene ring with hydroxyl group(s) and a hydrophobic moiety and are amphiphilic. Due to the amphiphilic properties, these molecules can incorporate into the phospholipid bilayers of cell membranes and interact with membranous structures, as well as hydrophobic domains of proteins. These interactions are nonspecific, and the action of phenolic lipids on a cell is comprehensive. No wonder that alkylresorcinols, the common representatives of phenolic lipids, do exert plural activities—antibacterial, antifungal, antiparasitic, anti-inflammatory, anticancer, and others—on diverse organisms and have attracted great attention. References to reviews on the history, occurrence, chemistry, and activities of phenolic lipids (e.g., by Kozubek and Tyman 1999 and Stasiuk and Kozubek 2010) can be found in the bibliography sections in this the book.

Plant and microbial alkylresorcinols are often regarded as secondary metabolites with a less important role in cellular physiology and biochemistry of the organism that produces them. Among bacteria, phenolic lipids were first described by Bu'Lock and Hudson in 1969 as components in leprosy mycobacterium, and later in cells of *Azotobacter* and *Pseudomonas* bacteria by scientists from USSR, USA, and Poland. Why are these compounds necessary for the producer organism? The viewpoint about the passive role of alkylresorcinols as components in vegetative and dormant bacterial cells changed upon studies conducted since the 1970s by Soviet and Russian scientists under the leadership of Prof. G.I. El-Registan. These studies demonstrated that several bacterial species synthesize extracellular autoregulatory factors, as mixture of alkylresorcinols' isomers and homologs, as well as other alkylated aromatic molecules, which control the development of a bacterial culture by causing growth arrest, deceleration of metabolic activity, and entrance to the dormant state. So, it is an oversimplification that bacterial phenolic lipids are secondary: they are synthesized at early growth stages, accumulate in cells and surrounding medium, redistribute, and are important for the acquirement of dormancy and stress resistance. These studies provided deep insight into nonspecific action of phenolic lipids and their synthetic analogs on different molecular, supramolecular, and cell targets. All these issues are discussed in this book.

The author of this book and the colleagues undertook long-standing studies focused on biomedical applications of phenolic lipids, particularly 4-hexylresorcinol chosen for the following reasons. This compound is available from companies in contrast to other alkylresorcinols with long aliphatic chain. Hexylresorcinol is used in cosmetics and medicine, or as a food additive and is not of toxicological concern at therapeutic doses. Another attractive property is the antitumor effect of 4-hexylresorcinol as reported by Japanese scientists in 1990. Most importantly, preceding studies in chemistry, biochemistry, and biology greatly inspired the author to initiate the experiments with 4-hexylresorcinol on different cell lines and biomaterials. Through literature reviews and the recent experimental findings, this book aims to illuminate the potential and seemingly unexpected applications of 4-hexylresorcinol. The Nature has been inventing numerous bioactive molecules, and their usefulness is still to be explored.

Russian Academy of Sciences
Moscow, Russia

Andrey Mulyukin

Preface

Since Stanley Miller's groundbreaking experiments, the scientific community has been fascinated with the chemical origins of life. Life depends on energy acquired through chemical dissociation. High-energy chemicals release energy by breaking chemical bonds, which is then used to power vital functions. Prokaryotes generate energy through metabolism of nutrients, while eukaryotes, with their more complex cellular organelles, require greater amounts of energy. As a result, eukaryotes need a dedicated power source, such as mitochondria, which reside within eukaryotic cells. Mitochondria metabolize glucose supplied by cellular receptors provided by the host cell, allowing them to access glucose without significant competition within the cytoplasm. Reactive oxygen species (ROS) are metabolic byproducts of mitochondria, which can be processed by the mitochondria themselves or other enzymes within the cytoplasm. Barring excessive glucose intake, this symbiotic relationship is generally harmonious.

However, not all cellular interactions result in positive outcomes. Mitochondria are semi-independent and their proliferation is regulated by the nucleus of differentiated cells through apoptotic signals. Cancer cells require substantial energy and consequently inhibit apoptotic signals, allowing for uncontrolled mitochondrial proliferation. Inhibiting mitochondrial respiration could therefore prove disastrous for cancer cells.

Traditional antimicrobial agents are ineffective against mitochondria due to their high toxicity. A safer approach to controlling mitochondrial activity involves studying microbial dormancy. Microorganisms often enter a dormant state to survive harsh conditions, which can be induced by small organic chemicals known as chaperones. These chemicals bind to proteins and stabilize their structure, restricting metabolic activity without causing cell death. Chaperones are less toxic than bactericidal agents and are produced by microorganisms themselves.

Interestingly, these chemicals have a broad spectrum of activity and can affect various species, including humans. Reducing mitochondrial respiration has diverse effects, such as promoting cellular differentiation. If the treatment goal involves cellular differentiation, chaperone-based agents may prove beneficial. Additionally, these chemicals can aid cellular survival by suppressing metabolic demand and promoting angiogenesis, making them particularly useful in tissue regeneration.

Numerous microorganisms and plants produce chaperones, offering a wide array of candidates for study. One such compound, resorcinolic lipid, is derived from plants. This book focuses extensively on the biomedical applications of 4-hexylresorcinol (4HR), a type of resorcinolic lipid. Already used in clinical trials, 4HR has applications as an antiseptic, food additive, and cosmetic ingredient. Apart from transient irritation of mucous membranes, 4HR has not been linked to severe complications. Through literature reviews and recent experimental findings, this book aims to illuminate further potential applications of 4HR.

In acknowledgment, I am grateful to research assistants Dr. Andrey Mulyukin, Dr. Chang-Hoon Chae, and Prof. Je-Yong Choi, colleagues at Gangneung-Wonju National University, authors, and researchers whose work has been referenced, Springer for their support, friends and family, and my father for their contributions to this book. This study has been worked with the support of a research grant of Gangneung-Wonju National University in 2022.

Gangneung, Kangwon-do, Korea (Republic of) Seong-Gon Kim

Contents

About the Author

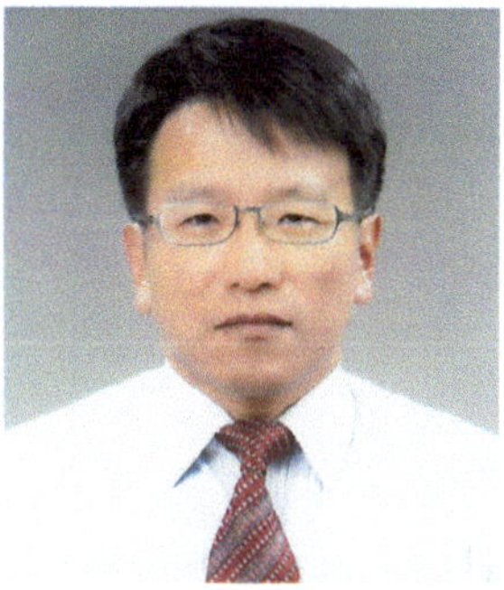

Seong-Gon Kim is a distinguished Professor at the Department of Oral and Maxillofacial Surgery, School of Dentistry, Gangneung-Wonju National University, Republic of Korea. With a dental degree and a Ph.D. from Seoul National University, Dr. Kim has forged an illustrious career, marked by significant academic and professional achievements. His expertise is rooted in oral pathology, and he has held various esteemed positions, including a Fellowship at Seoul National University Hospital and an Instructor role at Hallym University.

Dr. Kim's scholarly contributions are substantial, having authored numerous influential publications in international journals. His research spans a wide range of topics in oral and maxillofacial surgery, demonstrating his commitment to advancing the field. As an Editor-in-Chief and a member of various editorial committees, he has significantly influenced academic discourse. His dedication to his field is further exemplified by his role as Vice President of the Korean Society of Sericultural Science since 2021.

Chapter 1
Historical Background of Hexylresorcinol Research

Abstract This chapter outlines the reasons for investigating 4-hexylresorcinol (4HR). Originally synthesized as an antiseptic, Russian scientists discovered that it could also induce microbial dormancy. Additionally, 4HR has been shown to affect cancer cells in ways like microbial dormancy, leading to increased differentiation and decreased proliferation. The author explores 4HR's potential use in silk fibroin-based bone grafts and membranes as an antiseptic agent, as well as its potential in treating diabetes mellitus and promoting wound healing. Ultimately, this chapter emphasizes the versatility and minimal off-target effects of chemical chaperones like 4HR, which can have multiple therapeutic targets. Future research should focus on determining optimal therapeutic dosages and investigating the underlying mechanisms of 4HR's effects.

Keywords 4-hexylresorcinol (4HR) · Microbial dormancy · Cancer cells · Chemical chaperones · Cellular differentiation

4-Hexylresorcinol (4HR) is a synthetic resorcinolic lipid [1]. Kozubek and Tyman published a comprehensive review on resorcinolic lipids [2]. In the nature, there are many kinds of resorcinolic lipids (Fig. 1.1a). They are synthesized by the plants and the microorganisms, but mainly produced by the plants [2]. The firstly identified resorcinolic lipid was from plant (*Ginkgo biloba*) [3]. As common chemical backbone, a resorcinolic lipid has a hydroxyl-benzene and alkyl groups (Fig. 1.1). 4HR also has two hydroxyl groups and hexyl group (Fig. 1.1b). Because of two hydroxyl groups, 4HR has hydrophilic property, and these groups can be used for chelating ions. As hydrophobic moiety, 4HR has six carbon alkyl group. Some enzymes have five to six carbon-length hydrophobic domain as substrate-binding sitc. Whcn 4HR binds to this domain, it may have influence on the enzymatic activity [4, 5].

S.-G. Kim, *Biomedical Application of 4-Hexylresorcinol*,
https://doi.org/10.1007/978-981-97-0637-2_1

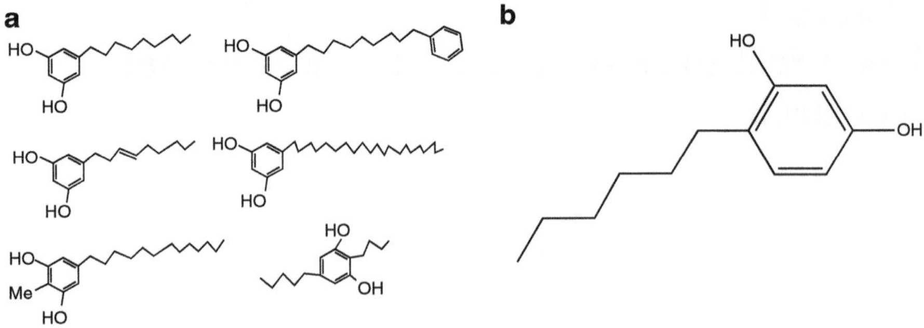

Fig. 1.1 Chemical structure resorcinolic lipids. (**a**) Some samples of known resorcinolic lipids. (**b**) Chemical structure of 4-hexylresorcinol. All resorcinolic lipids have common motif that is dihydroxyl benzene. The difference is an attached alkyl group

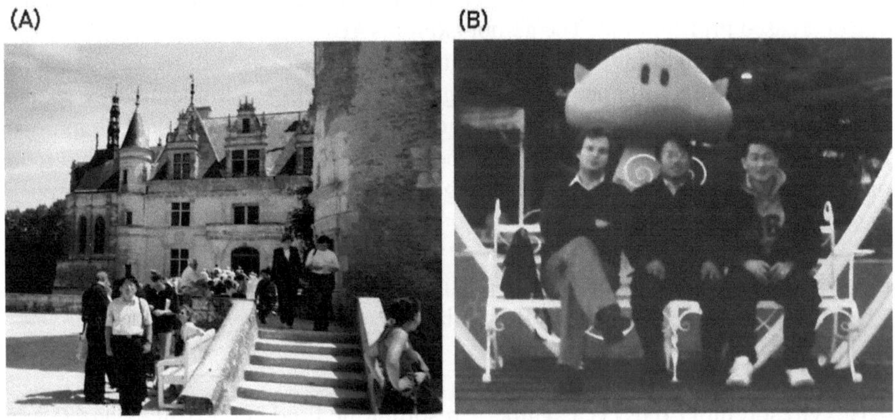

Fig. 1.2 Conference and meeting. (**a**) Conference in Blois, June 2000. (**b**) Dr. Mulyukin (left) visiting Korea in November 2001. Dr. Chae (right) and I (center) helped with his experiment on SCC-9 cells

1.1 Introduction of Hexylresorcinol

For me, 4HR was firstly introduced in 2000 by microbiologist, Dr. Mulyukin, who then worked in the laboratory of the brilliant scientist, Prof. El-Registan, Institute of Microbiology, Russian Academy of Sciences, Moscow. In June 2000, there was a Scientific meeting in Blois, France (XIIth "Recontres de Blois", Château de Blois, France; June 25–July 1, 2000). Many featured scientists had attended in this conference (Fig. 1.2a). Most featured figure was Stanley Miller, who performed the classic experiment for abiogenesis [6]. As he was quite old at that time, I had no any chance to discuss with him. In addition, Baruch Blumberg, Frank Drake, William Gilbert, et al. had attended that meeting, and I enjoyed active discussion with Dr. Gilbert.

There were many wonderful lectures that I did not want to lose. Dr. Mulyukin presented his topic entitled, “Resting Microbial Forms. Dormancy Inducing Autoregulatory Factors” [7]. He called 4HR as an alkyl hydroxy benzene (AHB). Though Miller amino acids were interesting issue, I was particularly interested in Dr. Mulyukin’s presentation. I felt that the discussion during the conference was not enough. Accordingly, I invited him several times to visit Korea and asked lectures. We had performed anticancer experiment using 4HR and SCC-9 cells (human tongue cancer cell) in Daejeon, Korea (Fig. 1.2b). He kindly shared his presentations that were presented in Korea. Some photos in this chapter are from his presentations.

There are many kinds of environmental stress. They are high/low temperature, radiation, starvation, dehydration, etc. When microorganisms receive the environmental stress, they should respond to the stress. If the stress is too strong, a part of microbial population will die. Another part may transform to a state of dormancy and survive. There can be several conditions for the dormancy transformation (Fig. 1.3). Growing microorganism should recognize the environmental change. In response to a stress, microbial cells may produce and/or release small molecules, so-called chemical chaperones. They also can be released from lysed cells. The diffused chemical chaperone can influence adjacent microorganisms. When a microbial cell receives the chemical chaperone, it can be either dying or dormant, depending on its concentration (Fig. 1.3).

By that time, dormancy-inducing autoregulatory factors in bacteria had been identified as different analogs and homologs of resorcinolic lipids [7], but they are commonly produced in very low amounts. Therefore, it is impossible to get such substances in quantities enough for vast experiments with a plenty of biological objects. Dr. Mulyukin told me at once that a ton of culture liquid (where cells grew)

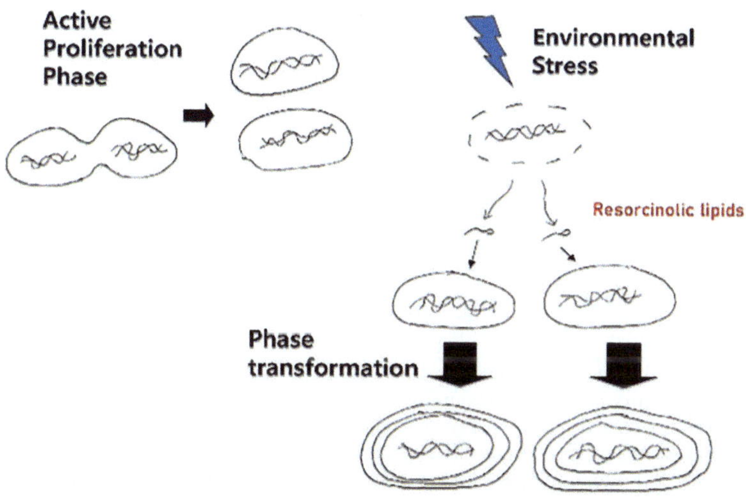

Fig. 1.3 A scheme of transformation. Resorcinolic lipids that are released from cells can trigger active-to-dormant state transformation

should be processed to produce about 1 g of a pure substance. Of course, this valuable substance was used for the basic experiments. In addition and then separately, commercially available analogs with the similar, not obligatorily exact, structure can be tested, and this was 4HR. Artificial synthesis of 4HR can be achieved from 3,5-dimethoxy benzaldehyde/3,5-dimethoxy benzylic alcohol/3,5-dimethoxy phenol [2]. Resorcinolic lipid in the living cell is considered as "secondary metabolite" [2]. The glucose is a metabolic precursor for the synthesis of 5-n-alkylresorcinol [2]. In case of long-chain resorcinolic lipid, the precursors are phospholipid and triglyceride, which are the components of the cellular membrane [2]. The intracellular compartment for the synthesis of resorcinolic lipid has been investigated. In case of plants, the resorcinolic lipid is synthesized in the chloroplast and etioplast membrane [2]. As these kinds of chemicals are produced during environmental stress and help the plant and microorganism to resist the stress, these chemicals can be called as "chemical chaperone" [8]. 4HR is considered as "chemical chaperone" and affects many enzymes and structural protein in the cell [8]. Recently, these chemical chaperones have been considered for treating disease. In this case, this type of chemical chaperone can be called as "pharmacologic chaperone" [9].

There are several key features in the microbial dormancy. First, the metabolic rate is extremely low and may not be detectable. As with aerobic bacteria, the level of oxygen consumption is closely associated with cellular metabolism (Fig. 1.4). Dormant cells

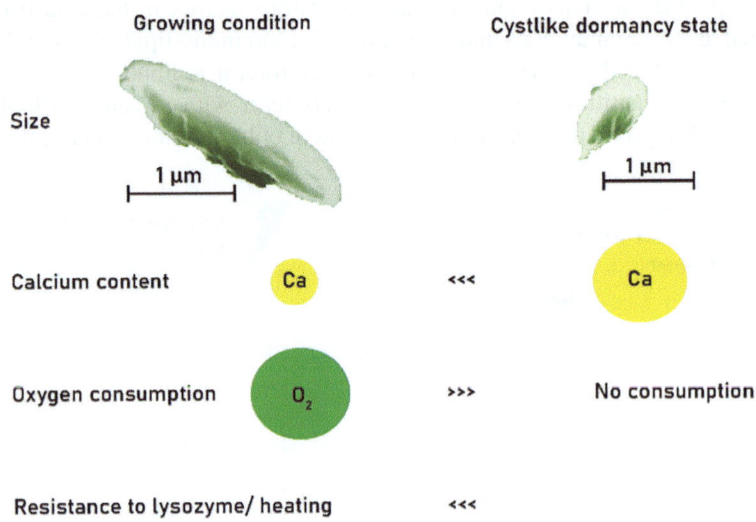

Fig. 1.4 The cystlike dormancy state exhibits certain distinctive characteristics. In the case of *Arthrobacter globiformis*, when its respiratory activity is compared to the growing condition, the cyst-like dormancy state displays no oxygen consumption. Additionally, it has been observed that cyst-like dormant *Micrococcus luteus* displays a higher resistance to lysozyme compared to the growing type [10]. Furthermore, a comprehensive investigation employing comparative scanning electron microscopy integrated with X-ray microanalysis has been conducted on individual microbial cells in different physiological states [11]. Notably, the cyst-like dormancy state exhibits significantly higher calcium content compared to the growing condition

showed no oxygen uptake as compared to growing one [10]. Dormant microbial cells are more resistant than active cells to enzymatic attack and heating [10].

The second feature is improving the structural stability of key proteins and DNA. Radiation and high/low temperature are extreme environmental stress. This type of stress is frequently observed in the nature. Many proteins have fragile structure and can be easily denatured by heating or radiation. As these molecules are fundamental elements in the life, their degradation should be prevented via structural stabilization. Another important feature of dormant cyst-like state in many microorganisms is that the cell wall becomes thicker and affords an additional protection [10].

Most interesting part for me was the species nonspecific effect of autoregulatory dormancy-inducing resorcinolic lipids and their analog—4HR [8, 12]. This means that their effect on a species A is similar effect with respect to a species B. At the end of Dr. Mulyukin's lecture, I raised my hand for a question, whether the application of resorcinolic lipid gave similar results in eukaryotic cells, too. He replied that it was quite possible and even predictable although he worked mainly with prokaryotes (bacteria). Soon after the meeting in Blois, the publication of several scientific teams, including Dr. Mulyukin and Prof. El-Registan, on the model of *ras*-transformed fibroblasts appeared and pointed to this possibility [8]. When transformed fibroblasts cultured in the nutrient supplied medium, they can proliferate. When 4HR is applied into the fibroblasts under the favorable environment, these fibroblasts decrease their proliferation and reduced their metabolism dose-dependently [8]. In detail, 4HR at concentration below 0.01 μM has no effect, but cellular division and metabolic activity are reversibly decreased at 0.01–10 μM, 4HR [8]. When culture medium is replaced by fresh, 4HR-free one, fibroblasts regain their metabolic activity. High dosage of 4HR can attenuate the stress from toxic reagent, too [8]. Interestingly, transformed fibroblasts by 4HR pretreatment change their morphology. There is no cell-to-cell contact and decreased cellular diameter with round shape [8]. This are similar morphological changes observed in dormant microbial cells (Fig. 1.4).

If 4HR has the species nonspecific effect, what will be its effect on the human? To answer this question, I should understand the equivalent physiological state to the microbial dormancy in the human. However, humans do not undergo dormancy. Considering that a human is a collection of different cellular types, the translation of microbial dormancy can be different to the cell types and their physiological state. If the cells are already in the terminal differentiation state and have no proliferating potential, they will be small difference in the microbial dormancy in terms of metabolic state. As these cells don't have a potential of resurrection, they are different from the dormancy. The administration of 4HR on these cells will be little effect because of their low metabolic rate. However, cancer cells are different from the terminally differentiated cells. They keep high metabolic state and proliferating potentials. Though I didn't know the dormancy in the cancer cells, the species nonspecific effect of 4HR might be helpful to control the human cancer growth. Accordingly, my research associated with 4HR had been focused on its anticancer effect. This research had been done intensively between 2001 and 2009.

1.2 Lessons from Microbial Dormancy for the Human

After the first meeting with Dr. Mulyukin in 2000, I wanted to test these microbial regulators in the oral cancer cells but had not found any way to get them. Historically, microbial dormancy regulators were called in publications as "*d1* factor," that is, a mixture of resorcinoilic or phenolic lipis with the target effect, or C_6-AHB, as synthesized. I asked him to help with this chemical for our cowork, and he advised me to purchase 4HR from Sigma-Aldrich.

Our first experiment was that the effect of 4HR administration on the mitochondrial respiration activity of SCC-9 (Fig. 1.5). They were measured using microculture tetrazolium (MTT) assay. NADH-dependent cellular enzymes are important in the oxidative metabolism, and these enzymes can reduce the tetrazolium dye. He observed the change after 4HR administration at 6 h and 40 h as early and late responses (Fig. 1.5). As we expected, the administration of 4HR (50–250 μM) decreased the activity of NADH-dependent cellular enzymes as time- and dose-dependent manner.

However, there are many potential anticancer reagents that are effective in the cellular experiments only. Therefore, the experiments on xenograft model were required to confirm. As I did not have any grant at that time, I could not perform the xenograft experiment until December 2003. Dr. Chae, who had worked in the Korea Research Institute of Bioscience and Biotechnology, helped me with this experiment (Fig. 1.2b). We performed this experiment between December 2003 and January 2004 (Fig. 1.6a). The administration route for 4HR to the animal was intraperitoneal injection.

The administered dosage was referenced from other experiments. Three different dosage groups were tested (1, 10, and 100 mg/kg of 4HR). 4HR was administered daily via intraperitoneal injection as predetermined dosage. Unfortunately, the

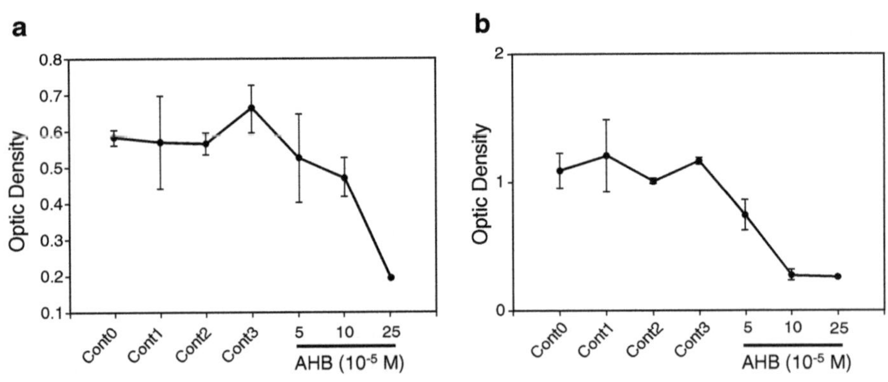

Fig. 1.5 MTT assay for SCC-9 cells after 4HR treatment. Mulyukin performed the experiment for the control for four times. (**a**) The observation at 6 h after 4HR administration. The optic density (OD) value was lower in the groups administered 4HR as dose-dependently. (**b**) The observation at 40 h after 4HR administration. Similar pattern was observed for those at 6 h

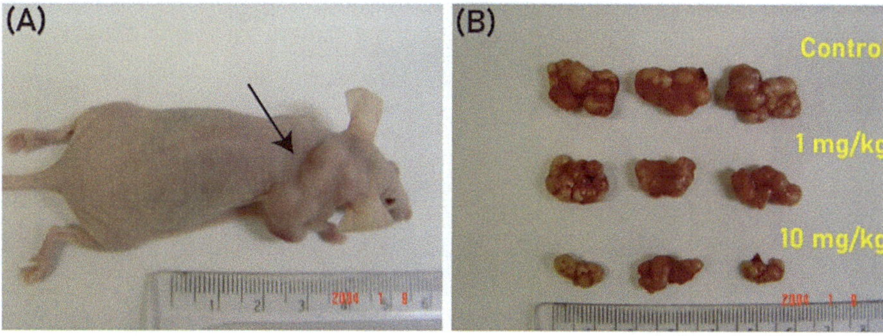

Fig. 1.6 Xenograft of SCC-9 cells in the back skin of nude mice. (**a**) Tumor mass (arrow) was clearly identified in the control group. (**b**) The enucleated tumor mass from each animal at 16 days after initial 4HR administration. The average size of tumor mass was significantly smaller in 4HR groups compared to those in control group ($P < 0.05$)

animals that received 100 mg/kg of 4HR were dead on the second day of the administration. The reduction of tumor size was evident in 1 and 10 mg/kg of 4HR groups compared to the control group (Fig. 1.6b).

The translation of microbial dormancy in the eukaryote was difficult. Considering several features of microbial dormancy such as relatively reduced growth and metabolism, the dormant cancer cells mimic non-cancer cells. They might show higher level of differentiation and lower mitotic rate than untreated control. Keratin is well-known differentiation marker for the epithelial cells. As SCC-9 cell is originated from squamous epithelial cell of the tongue, if SCC-9 is differentiated by 4HR administration, the expression level of keratin should be increased. Ki67 is a marker for cellular proliferation. Thus, the expression pattern of Ki67 should be opposite to that of keratin after 4HR administration (Fig. 1.7).

From these experiments, 4HR-induced changes in oral cancer cells had been clearly identified. However, detailed mechanism was unclear until 2009. We found that certain groups of transcription factors are influenced by 4HR administration. Detailed anticancer mechanism of 4HR will be shown in Chap. 3. Though there remain many steps to unveil full story, we had a lot of achievements for decades.

I received the first grant from Korean government for the development of silk fibroin-based bone graft material from 2009. As silk fibroin has low toxicity and provides cellular attachment on its surface, microorganism in the oral cavity may attach to the silk graft easily and induce inflammation. 4HR is well known antiseptic [13]. Thus, 4HR incorporation into the silk fibroin-based graft may be helpful for preventing infection. However, our calvarial defect model was not proper to test this hypothesis even we did the graft contamination with oral microflora. This model just provided the information of comparative bone formation ability of 4HR-incorporated graft (Fig. 1.8). Without adding calcium, silk fibroin protein plus 4HR did not induce successful bone formation in our animal model. Though the silk fibroin-based bone graft was disappointing, the silk fibroin-based membrane for

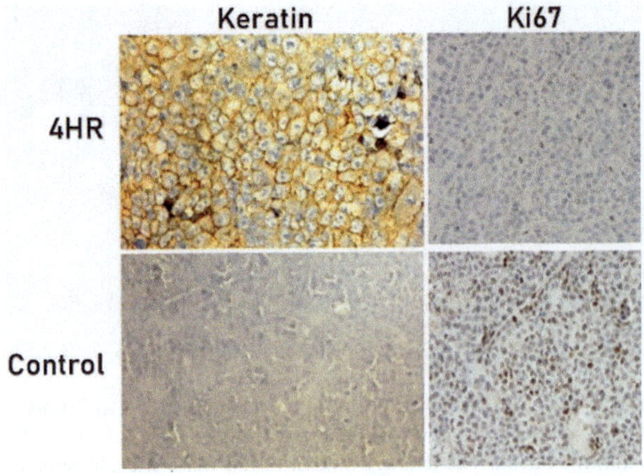

Fig. 1.7 Immunohistochemistry for the specimens from xenograft of SCC-9 cells. The expression level of keratin was higher in 4HR group. However, the expression level of Ki67 was higher in the control group (original magnification ×100, counterstained with Mayer's haematoxylin)

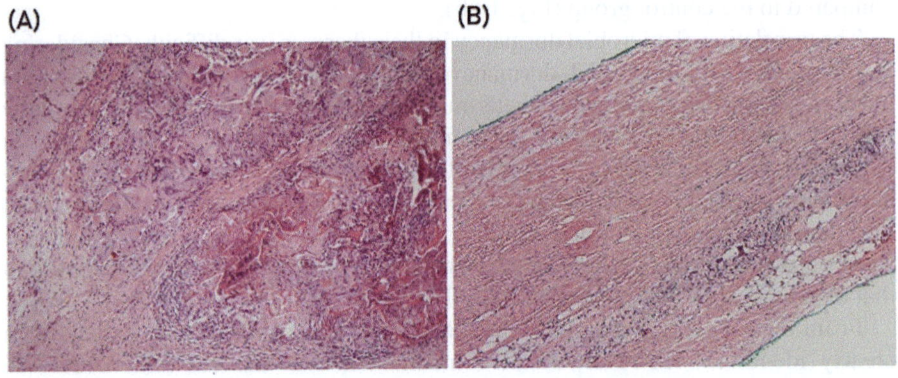

Fig. 1.8 The silk fibroin-based bone grafts were applied into the calvarial defect of the rabbits. The silk-based grafts were contaminated with *Acinetobacter actinomycetemcomitans,* which is well-known oral microflora and responsible for periodontitis. There were two groups of graft. They are the silk fibroin only (**a**) and 4HR-incorporated silk fibroin (**b**). The specimens were taken at 8 weeks later surgery. In case of silk fibroin only group, chronic inflammation with residual graft was found (**a**). However, 4HR-incorporated silk fibroin group showed fibrotic tissue without residual graft (**b**) (original magnification ×100, stained with haematoxylin and eosin)

guided bone regeneration was excellent [14]. In addition, I found that 4HR-incorporated silk fibroin graft showed less foreign body reaction and rapid degradation of graft (Fig. 1.8). These findings were hints for the development of biodegradable silk suture [15]. While investigating its mechanism, I found that 4HR is M2 polarizing agent for tissue resident macrophage. The effect of 4HR on wound healing and tissue engineering will be discussed in Chaps. 6 and 7.

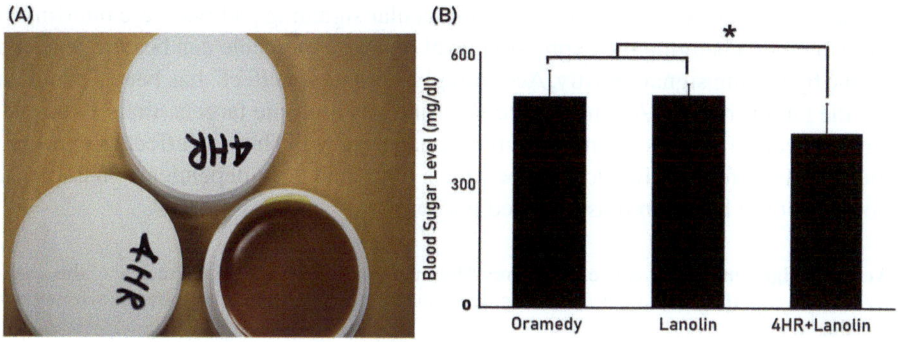

Fig. 1.9 The effect of 4HR ointment on the intraoral ulcer in DM animal model. (**a**) 4HR ointment based on lanolin oil. (**b**) The blood sugar level in the fasting condition. It was significantly lower in 4HR group compared to commercially available intraoral ointment (Oramedy®) and lanolin base only group (*$P < 0.05$)

As shown above, there is close relation between cellular metabolism and 4HR application. Diabetes is a representative human metabolic disease. The complications associated with diabetes mellitus (DM) are associated with inflammation caused by metabolic imbalance. Considering that 4HR has the species nonspecifically decreasing metabolism effect, the application of 4HR might be helpful in managing DM-associated complications. As my profession is an oral and maxillofacial surgeon, I have faced many DM patients having difficulty in the postoperative wound management.

Lanolin-based 4HR ointment has been widely studied to accelerate wound healing in our lab (Fig. 1.9a). The application of 4HR ointment could increase bone density in the arthritic knee joint animal model (personal communication with Choi JY in Kyungpook National University). Its application on intra-oral ulcer might show its therapeutic effect. In case of intra-oral ulcer animal model, most challenging part of study design was too rapid healing to observe the difference among groups. As DM is associated with delayed wound healing, we designed buccal mucosal ulcer model in the DM animal. During our investigation of intra-oral ulcer healing by 4HR ointment application in this model, we found that the blood sugar level was lowered in 4HR group (Fig. 1.9b). From this observation, the effect of 4HR on the attenuating DM complications had been widely studied. It will be discussed in Chap. 8.

1.3 Closing Remarks

A group of proteins is involved in the phase transformation from the active proliferating to the inactive state. The chemical chaperone is a key element for this phase transformation. This is the main difference between the chemical chaperone and the drug for target therapy. The drug for the target therapy is aimed to change specific intracellular signaling pathway. However, there are multiple targets for the chemical chaperone. The main purpose of the chemical chaperone application is the changing intracellular metabolic balance. As the molecular signaling pathways are interlinked to each other, changing the expression level of single molecule can be compensated by the bypassing signal, mostly. Accordingly, "off-target effect" has been a problem for the target therapy. As chemical chaperone has multiple targets, there is no off-target effect. The application of chemical chaperone will show its effect as expected mostly. The effect of chemical chaperone is time- and dose-dependent. Therapeutic dosage should be tailored as intended purpose.

Acknowledgments I appreciate Dr. Andrey Mulyukin for his extremely kind review of this chapter and for providing important figures. In addition, this project could not be started without our meeting in France.

References

1. Leonard V (1925) The significance of hexylresorcinol and its homologues in relation to the problem of internal antisepsis. Science 62(1610):408–412
2. Kozubek A, Tyman JH (1999) Resorcinolic lipids, the natural non-isoprenoid phenolic amphiphiles and their biological activity. Chem Rev 99:1–26
3. Amico V, Biondi D, Cunsolo F et al (1990) Three Acetogenins from the Brown alga Caulocystis cephalornithos. J Nat Prod 53(5):1379–1382
4. Belousova L, Lozinsky V, Vainerman E et al (1989) In: Debabov VG (ed) Fermenty Mikroorganizmov (enzymes of microorganisms). VNIISENTI, Moscow, p 224
5. Kim JY, Kweon HY, Kim DW et al (2021) 4-hexylresorcinol inhibits class I histone deacetylases in human umbilical cord endothelial cells. Appl Sci 11(8):3486
6. Miller SL (1953) A production of amino acids under possible primitive earth conditions. Science 117(3046):528–529
7. Mulyukin AL, Suzina NS, Duda VI, Kolpakov AN, Ilinskaya ON, El-Registan GI (2000) Resting microbial forms. Dormancy inducing autoregulatory factors. Frontiers of life, proceedings of the XIIth Recontres de Blois, pp 145–151
8. Il'inskaya ON, Kolpakov AI, Mulyukin AL et al (2000) Effect of membrane-active microbial autoregulators on the growth of cultured ras-transformed fibroblasts. Appl Biochem Microbiol 36:473–477
9. Kim SG (2022) 4-hexylresorcinol: pharmacologic chaperone and its application for wound healing. Maxillofac Plast Reconstr Surg 44:5
10. El-Registan GI, Mulyukin AL, Nikolaev YA et al (2005) The role of microbial low-molecular-weight autoregulatory factors (alkylhydroxybenzenes) in resistance of microorganisms to radiation and heat shock. Adv Space Res 36(9):1718–1728
11. Mulyukin A, Sorokin V, Loiko N et al (2002) Comparative study of the elemental composition of vegetative and resting microbial cells. Microbiology 71(1):37–48
12. Mulyukin A, Demkina E, Kozlova A et al (2001) Synthesis of anabiosis autoinducers by non-spore-forming bacteria as a mechanism regulating their activity in soil and subsoil sedimentary rocks. Microbiology 70:535–541
13. Evans R, Baker P, Coburn R et al (1977) In vitro antiplaque effects of antiseptic phenols. J Periodontol 48(3):156–162
14. Lee SW, Kim SG (2014) Membranes for the guided bone regeneration. Maxillofac Plast Reconstr Surg 36(6):239
15. Jo YY, Kweon H, Kim DW et al (2017) Accelerated biodegradation of silk sutures through matrix metalloproteinase activation by incorporating 4-hexylresorcinol. Sci Rep 7:42441

Chapter 2
4-Hexylresorcinol: Antiseptic, Cosmetics, and Food Industry

Abstract 4-Hexylresorcinol (4HR) is a versatile compound with a range of applications in cosmetics, food preservation, antiseptics, anthelmintics, and lozenges. In cosmetics, it has antiaging, anti-inflammatory, and anti-pigmentation properties. As a food additive, 4HR's tyrosinase inhibition properties can extend food storage time, but its safety and potential estrogenic effects need further evaluation. Although it was originally developed as an antiseptic, 4HR's antibacterial and antifungal properties are weaker compared to alternative substances. Its anthelmintic potential is limited, with more effective alternatives available. However, 4HR has demonstrated notable virucidal effects and pain-relief properties when used in lozenges for sore throat treatment. Despite the potential benefits, 4HR's effectiveness in certain applications is overshadowed by alternative substances, and its role as a histone deacetylase inhibitor warrants further investigation for possible use in nutraceuticals. Overall, the diverse applications of 4HR highlight its potential across various industries, but more research is needed to fully understand its implications and limitations.

Keywords 4-hexylresorcinol (4HR) · Cosmetics · Food preservation · Tyrosinase inhibition · Antiseptic · Lozenges

Chaperones are synthesized in response to cellular crisis caused by environmental stress, with the aim of aiding cell survival. In humans, the heat shock protein (HSP) family serves as a molecular chaperone and is synthesized when cells receive an excessive amount of heat energy. HSP plays a crucial role in stabilizing structural proteins and preventing protein denaturation. Unlike some other chaperones, HSP is not specific to any single protein. As rescuing a single protein alone is insufficient for cell survival, any molecule considered a chaperone must have multiple targets.

4-Hexylresorcinol (4HR) is a chemical chaperone that can bind to multiple intracellular enzymes and impact their activity. While some enzymes experience an increase in activity with the application of 4HR, most exhibit a decrease. Notably, tyrosinase is one such enzyme that is strongly inhibited by 4HR. Tyrosinase is responsible for two steps in melanin synthesis, namely the hydroxylation of L-tyrosine and the enzymatic oxidation of L-DOPA (Fig. 2.1) [1]. Melanin provides

S.-G. Kim, *Biomedical Application of 4-Hexylresorcinol*,
https://doi.org/10.1007/978-981-97-0637-2_2

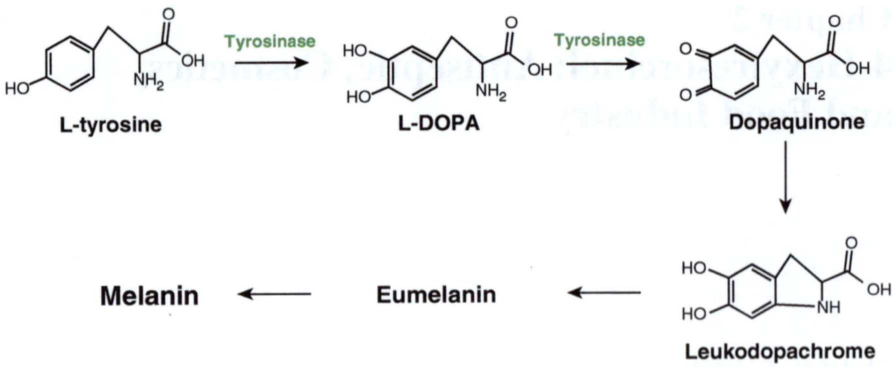

Fig. 2.1 The synthesis of melanin

protection against ultraviolet rays but is also a black pigment that some individuals may find undesirable in their skin or food. Consequently, the cosmetic and food industries have widely adopted 4HR for its commercial applications. Additionally, 4HR serves as a dormancy inducer as a chemical chaperone and can inhibit microbial proliferation, making it a commonly used antiseptic.

2.1 Hexylresorcinol in Cosmetics

The cosmetic industry places significant importance on treating excessive melanin pigmentation on the skin. The global market for skin lightening cosmetics was valued at approximately 23 billion US dollars in 2020, with market growth especially high in Asian and African regions. It is projected that these markets will reach 31.2 billion US dollars by 2024 [2, 3]. Approximately 28% of people worldwide use these types of cosmetics [4]. One common method for inhibiting melanin production is through tyrosinase inhibition [5].

Common formulations for anti-pigmentation cosmetics include creams, lotions, and soaps [6]. In the past, ingredients such as steroids, mercury, and hydroquinone were commonly used in these formulations [7]. However, long-term use of these chemicals may pose health risks [8, 9]. Phenolic compounds derived from plants are being explored as potential alternatives to these chemicals [10]. Compounds such as flavonoids and chalcones have demonstrated anti-tyrosinase activity [11]. One such phenolic compound is 4HR, which has been shown to inhibit tyrosinase and reduce melanin production in clinical trials [12, 13].

The composition for cosmetics containing 4HR has been patented [14, 15], and many commercial products now use 4HR as their main skin whitening ingredient due to its safety and strong tyrosinase inhibition properties (Table 2.1). Compared to other potential inhibitors, such as 4-butylresorcinol, 4-phenylethyl resorcinol, hydroquinone, Kojic acid, and arbutin, 4HR is the strongest tyrosinase inhibitor in terms of inhibition potency [16]. Use of 4HR-based cosmetics has been shown to

Table 2.1 Commercially available cosmetic products

Brand name	4HR concentration	Manufacturer	Indication
HYDRO BRIGHT TREATMENT 3	1%	Medature	An invigorating brightening treatment and pigment corrector
DEPI 50+	0.5%	Canova	Day cream with very high sun protection that prevents photo-induced hyperpigmentation
HXR-EYE CREAM	0.1%	Fillmed	A lightweight gel specially formulated for the sensitive eye area
Retinol & Hexylresorcinol Peel	Unidentified	Med Calia	An exfoliating formula for advanced aging signs

reduce facial wrinkles and melanin pigmentation [17]. When present with hydrogen peroxide or vitamin C, 4HR can also behave as a substrate of tyrosinase [18], suggesting that it may bind to the substrate-binding domain of tyrosinase.

The combination of 4HR and niacinamide has shown promising results in addressing hyperpigmentation and improving skin health. 4HR, known for its skin whitening properties, has been widely studied for its effectiveness in lightening skin tone [19]. While it can effectively target hyperpigmentation on its own, its effects may be amplified when combined with other active ingredients. Niacinamide, a common component in hyperpigmentation treatments, has been found to be particularly effective in regulating melanin production [19].

Studies have demonstrated that the combination of 4HR and niacinamide can lead to an increase in procollagen synthesis in dermal fibroblasts [16]. Collagen is essential for maintaining the firmness and elasticity of the skin, and increased procollagen synthesis can contribute to a more youthful and resilient complexion. This suggests that the synergistic effect between 4HR and niacinamide may not only improve skin color and reduce pigmentation but also enhance overall skin firmness [19].

Furthermore, the combination of 4HR and niacinamide has been shown to be more effective in achieving desired outcomes compared to niacinamide used alone [19]. Researchers have observed greater improvements in skin color and firmness when the two ingredients are combined, suggesting a potential additive or synergistic effect. These findings support the idea that coupling 4HR with niacinamide can enhance their individual benefits and provide superior results in addressing hyperpigmentation.

The United States has frequently used hydroquinone for the treatment of pigmented skin. However, a randomized prospective clinical trial comparing hydroquinone (2%) with 4HR (1%) demonstrated similar efficacy in reducing facial and hand pigmentation, with no reported adverse effects for topical application of 1% 4HR [20]. In addition, a combination of 4HR, silymarin, vitamins C and E applied to skin explants showed protection against UVB-induced inflammation and improved skin tone and color [21]. This combination has already been commercialized and is available in the market (Fig. 2.2).

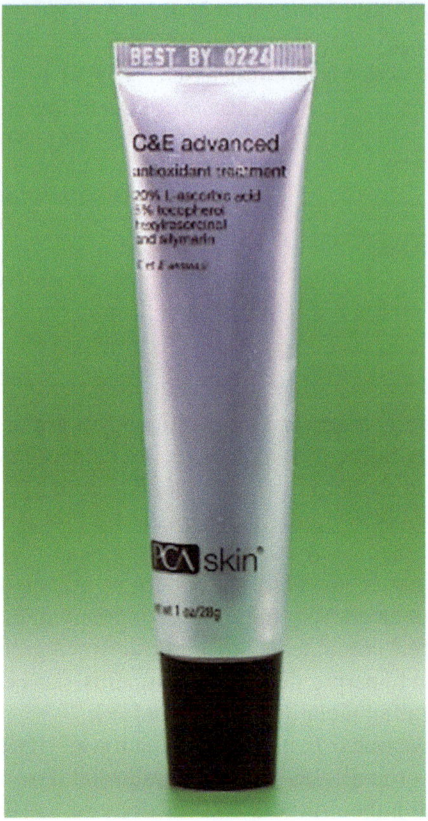

Fig. 2.2 4HR, silymarin, vitamin C and E combination

2.2 Hexylresorcinol in Food

The discoloration of food is a common indication of decreased freshness, leading to a loss in commercial value [22]. This phenomenon is particularly evident in fruits and shrimps, where melanin pigmentation plays a significant role, and the enzyme tyrosinase is primarily responsible for the color change [1, 23]. To combat this issue, the utilization of tyrosinase inhibitors has been widely adopted in the food industry to delay the color change and extend the storage time of foods [24].

Tyrosinase inhibitors can be classified into two categories: synthetic chemicals and natural products [25]. Although both types have been used in the food industry, safety concerns limit the use of only a few synthetic tyrosinase inhibitors. On the other hand, natural products offer the advantage of being safer. Nevertheless, extracting the active component from natural products often proves to be expensive and yields a low ratio [24]. Therefore, despite the potential benefits of using natural tyrosinase inhibitors in the food industry, their practical application is challenging due to cost and extraction limitations.

When considering the use of a tyrosinase inhibitor as a food additive, it is important to ensure that it is safe for consumption. This means that the inhibitor should not pose any harm if ingested. Additionally, it should not undergo any harmful chemical changes during the cooking process, which could potentially produce harmful by-products. The inhibitor should also not interfere with the digestion process of the food, as this could lead to gastrointestinal issues. Finally, if possible, the inhibitor should have minimal absorption through the gastrointestinal tract to prevent any potential systemic effects. Therefore, when selecting a tyrosinase inhibitor as a food additive, it is crucial to carefully evaluate its safety and potential effects on both the food and the consumer.

Numerous natural and synthetic phenolic compounds have been identified to have the ability to bind to the estrogen receptor (ER) and exhibit estrogenic activity [26]. These compounds, commonly referred to as xenoestrogens, have been defined by the European Commission as exogenous substances or mixtures that alter the functions of the endocrine system and cause adverse health effects in intact organisms or their offspring. However, it is important to note that mere binding affinity to the ER does not classify a compound as a xenoestrogen; it must also induce adverse health effects.

Phenolic compounds, such as 4HR, have the potential to bind to the ER and disrupt the normal functioning of the endocrine system [27]. Given that 4HR is used as a food additive, it is crucial to assess its potential estrogenic effects. Computational protein and ligand interaction models have indicated a high affinity of 4HR to the ER. However, the results of competition assays did not show any binding to the ER [27]. Interestingly, 4HR was found to be active in transactivation assays [27]. It is worth mentioning that these findings were obtained from cellular-level experiments, and the comprehensive understanding of the adverse health effects associated with 4HR is still lacking.

The previous publication highlights that although the binding affinity of 4HR to ER is weak, its application in MCF-7 cells at concentrations of 1–10 μM leads to an increased activity of oestrogen-responsive promoters [27]. This suggests that 4HR may have an indirect effect on ER signaling pathways or interact with other proteins involved in the regulation of these promoters. It is noteworthy that despite the widespread use of 4HR in various applications, there have been no reported adverse effects in clinical trials so far. This indicates that the potential weak binding affinity of 4HR to ER does not seem to have significant negative consequences in a clinical setting.

Animal studies have provided insights into the effects of 4HR on spermatogenesis. Administration of a lethal dose of 1 g/kg body weight/day of 4HR has been shown to decrease spermatogenesis [28]. However, this decrease might be attributed to the toxic effects of an extremely high dose rather than a direct effect of 4HR on spermatogenesis. In fact, there is evidence that administering 4HR can improve spermatogenesis in animal models with diabetes. This suggests that 4HR may have a complex relationship with spermatogenesis, and further research is required to fully understand its effects in different contexts.

Xenoestrogens are known to activate the growth of breast cancer cells, with bisphenol-A (BPA) being a well-known example [29]. However, when comparing the effects of 4HR and BPA on breast cancer cell growth, 4HR appears to exhibit the opposite behaviour to BPA. Unlike several other xenoestrogens, which increase ER activity in the absence of oestradiol, 4HR does not activate ER in this way [30]. The activation of ERα typically results in increased phosphorylation of extracellular signal-regulated kinase (ERK) [31], but while BPA application increases p-ERK1/2 expression, 4HR does not have this effect (as seen in Fig. 2.3).

Previous research has suggested that the systemic administration of 4HR, if it acts like a hormone, may lead to an increase in prolactin levels and the expression of ER in the pituitary gland. This effect seems to be particularly prominent in ovariectomy animal models, where decreased blood estrogen levels are observed [33]. Studies have also demonstrated that the administration of estrogen-like chemicals can enhance ER expression in the anterior pituitary gland and elevate serum prolactin levels [34].

In the ovariectomized model, it has been observed that the administration of oestradiol and BPA leads to an increase in serum prolactin levels as well as the expression levels of ERα, ERβ, and prolactin in the pituitary glands when compared

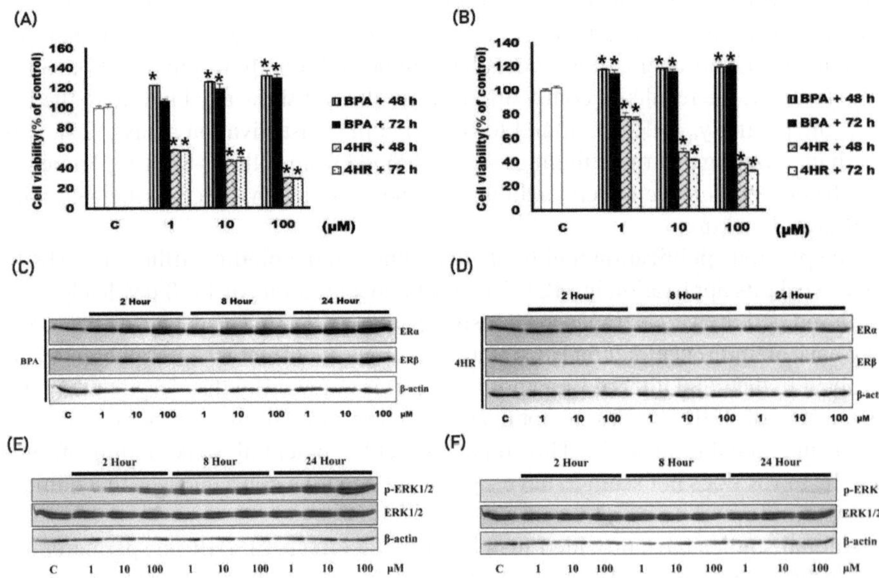

Fig. 2.3 Comparison the bioactivity between bisphenol A (BPA) and 4-hexylresorcinol (4HR). The application of BPA (1–100 μM) to MCF-7 cells (**a**) and SK-BR-3 cells (**b**) showed increased cell viability compared to solvent only group at 48 and 72 h after administration. However, the application of 4HR with the same range of concentration showed the opposite trend to BPA group (*$P < 0.05$). (**c**) The application of BPA increased the expression level of estrogen receptors (ERs). However, there is little change in ERs expression level after 4HR administration (**d**). The expression level of p-ERK1/2 is increased by BPA (**e**), but not by 4HR (**f**). (Original images have been published in author's article [32] and modified for this book)

to untreated controls (Fig. 2.4). However, in comparison to the untreated control group, the administration of 4HR did not affect serum prolactin levels and did not induce an increase in the expression levels of ER (Fig. 2.4). Furthermore, an examination of the uterine epithelium revealed that it was thicker in the estradiol groups compared to the 4HR and solvent-only groups (Fig. 2.4a).

These findings suggest that the effect of 4HR on prolactin levels and ER expression may differ from that of oestradiol and BPA in ovariectomy animal models. While the administration of 4HR did not appear to influence serum prolactin levels or ER expression, oestradiol and BPA demonstrated clear effects in increasing these parameters. The difference in uterine epithelial thickness between the groups further indicates the differential effects of these substances. These results highlight the importance of studying the specific mechanisms of action and potential hormonal effects of different chemicals, as their impacts may vary even within the same experimental model. Further research is warranted to elucidate the underlying mechanisms and consequences of 4HR administration in hormone regulation.

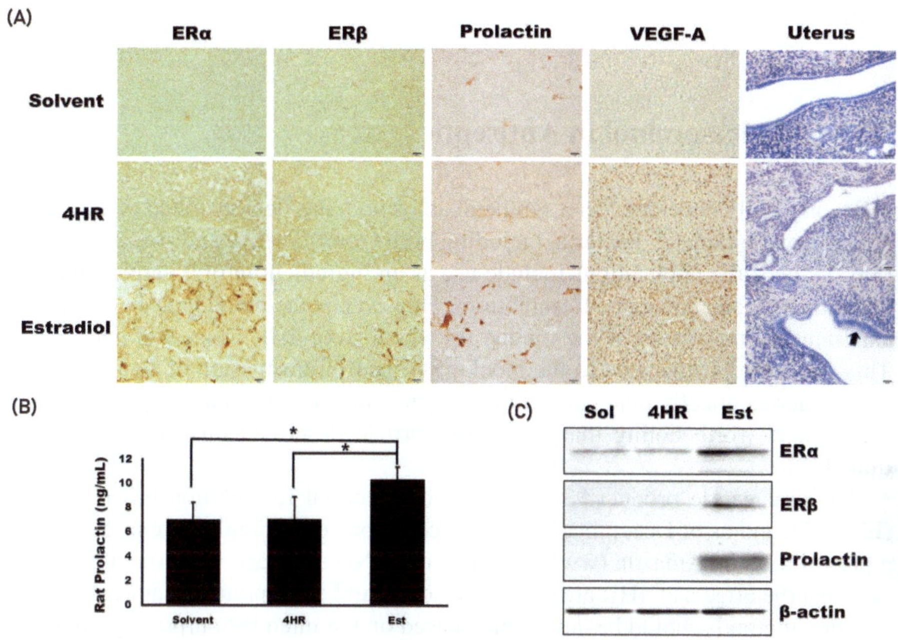

Fig. 2.4 The effect of 4-hexylresorcinol (4HR) administration on the ovariectomized animal model. (**a**) In the immunohistochemical study, the administration of estradiol increases the expression level of estrogen receptor-α (ERα), ERβ, prolactin, and vascular endothelial growth factor-A (VEGF-A) in the pituitary gland. The epithelial thickness of the uterus is also increased (arrow). Except for VEGF-A, the expression level of other markers in 4HR group is not much changed compared to those of solvent only group. (**b**) Serum prolactin level is significantly increased in estradiol group (Est) compared to the other groups (*$P < 0.05$). (**c**) Western blots for (ERα), ERβ, and prolactin are done for the protein extract from the pituitary gland. The results are in accord to those of immunohistochemistry. (Original images have been published in author's article [32] and modified for this book)

According to experimental research conducted on ovariectomized animals, it has been observed that 4-hydroxyresveratrol (4HR) does not exhibit estrogen-like effects but instead functions as a histone deacetylase inhibitor (HDACi) [32]. This mechanism of action results in the modulation of gene translation and protein expression levels. Because of such alterations in cellular processes, increased expression of the transforming growth factor-β family and subsequent upregulation of vascular endothelial growth factor (VEGF) occur. It is postulated that these molecular changes could contribute to calcification and angiogenesis, like the effects exerted by estrogen.

In relation to its potential application as a food additive for anti-browning purposes, it is noteworthy to mention that the availability of numerous alternative agents with the same functionality may render 4HR unsuitable for this specific application. Furthermore, it should be acknowledged that the effects of 4HR are influenced by the dosage and route of administration. Therefore, when considering the incorporation of 4HR as a food additive in nutraceuticals, it is crucial to tailor the dosage and administration method according to the intended purpose.

2.3 Hexylresorcinol in Antiseptic

4HR, originally developed as a synthetic antiseptic, has demonstrated effectiveness against a wide range of bacteria, including both Gram-positive and -negative strains [35]. Its versatile applications include use as an ingredient in oral gargles, humidifier additives, and antiseptic formulations. However, some individuals have reported experiencing numbness of the tongue tip when using 4HR as an oral gargle [36]. This sensation is attributed to the blocking of neurotransmission of sensory nerves and is therapeutically beneficial for managing sore throat, commonly seen in lozenges. It is worth noting that a previous article described this effect as "irritation" [37].

The oral gargle product "S.T.37" is a commercial formulation based on 4HR (Fig. 2.5), and as of December 7, 2022, it could be conveniently purchased without a prescription on Amazon (www.amazon.com). Nevertheless, it is crucial to recognize that the effects of 4HR are dose-dependent, and appropriate dosage and administration methods should be determined based on the intended purpose, particularly when used as a food additive in nutraceuticals.

The antimicrobial efficacy of the oral disinfectant "S.T.37" has been found to be comparatively weaker than that of hydrogen peroxide glycerite, as reported in a study [37]. Similarly, 4HR has been proposed as an air disinfectant [38]; however, a study conducted to evaluate its effectiveness in preventing the common cold through air disinfection provided no evidence to support its efficacy [39].

Regarding its efficacy as an antiplaque agent, it has been observed that 4HR does not integrate into the tooth surface [40]. Nevertheless, it has shown the ability to inhibit the formation of dental plaque in a dose- and time-dependent manner [41].

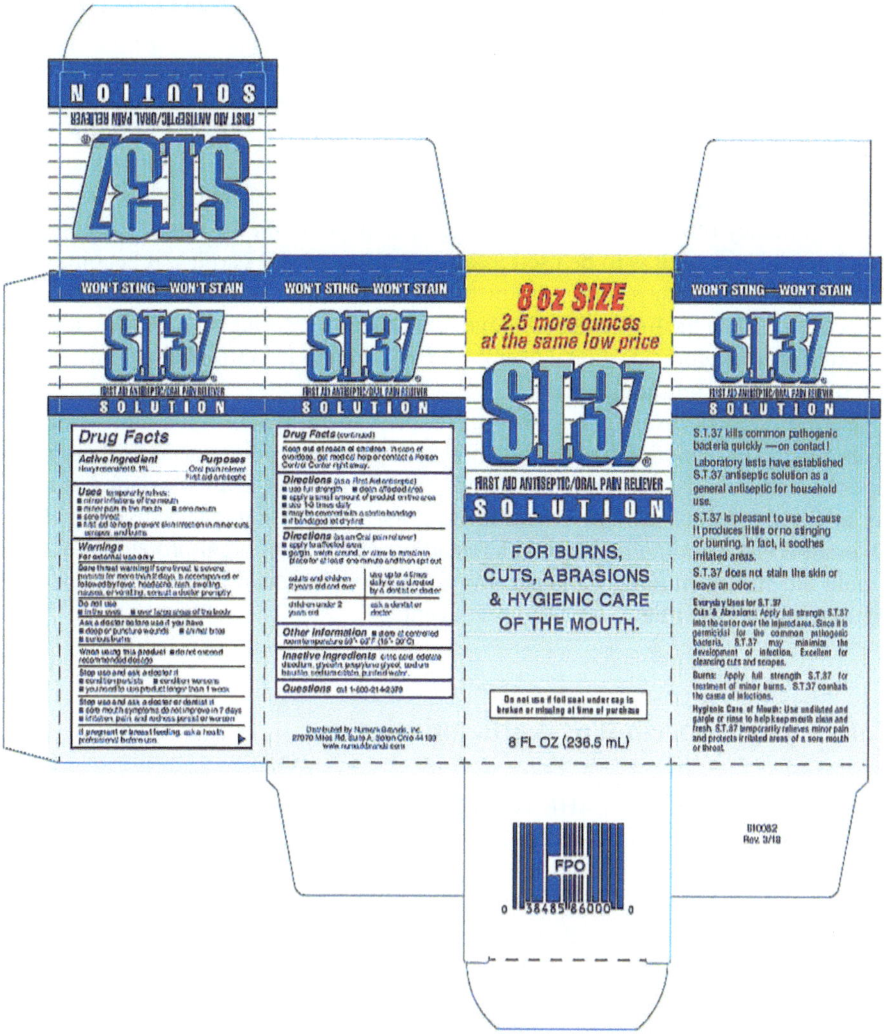

Fig. 2.5 The package for S.T.37

The effectiveness of 4HR in inhibiting bacterial growth has been demonstrated with an effective dose of 15 μg/mL and 24-h exposure required for 50% inhibition [41].

Given the weaker antibacterial effect of "S.T.37" compared to hydrogen peroxide glycerite, caution should be exercised when considering its use in situations requiring a more potent antimicrobial action. The lack of evidence supporting the efficacy of 4HR as an air disinfectant for preventing the common cold raises questions about its usefulness in combating respiratory infections. Despite not integrating into the tooth surface, 4HR has demonstrated effectiveness in inhibiting the formation of dental plaque. Further research is needed to explore the full potential of 4HR as an antiplaque agent and its optimal dosage and exposure time for greater inhibition of bacterial growth.

The antifungal properties of 4HR have not been extensively investigated within the scientific literature. However, acrisorcin, a derivative of 4HR, has been employed in the treatment of tinea versicolor at a concentration of 0.2% [42]. Despite this, it is worth noting that there exists a myriad of alternative compounds that exhibit potent antimicrobial effects, raising questions about the suitability of 4HR as an antiseptic agent.

The efficacy of 4HR appears to be highly dependent on the dosage and method of administration. If it is to be used as an ingredient in oral gargles, it becomes crucial to tailor the dosage and administration method to meet specific therapeutic objectives. Given the limited knowledge regarding its antifungal properties, it would be prudent to explore additional avenues of research to better understand the potential of 4HR as an antifungal agent.

Further studies investigating the antifungal capabilities of 4HR and its derivatives would be beneficial to establish its efficacy and potential as a therapeutic option. Additionally, comparative studies examining 4HR against existing antiseptic alternatives may provide valuable insights to guide clinical decision-making. Overall, a more comprehensive understanding of the antifungal properties of 4HR would aid in determining its suitability for various medical applications and thus optimizing its potential as an antiseptic agent.

2.4 Hexylresorcinol as Anthelmintics

The oral bioavailability of 4HR is generally low. However, this limitation can be advantageous in the context of helminth control, as it allows for the administration of high oral doses [43]. In adults, a dose of 1 g of encapsulated 4HR is commonly employed for anthelmintic treatment, primarily to minimize potential irritation to the buccal mucosa [43]. Another route of administration for 4HR is through inclusion in enema solutions, which are available for both animals and humans [44]. Clinical trials have shown that 4HR is effective against various types of parasitic worms, including roundworms, flukes, and tapeworms, in humans. The cure rate for ascariasis was reported at 66.6% with an egg reduction rate of 94%, although lower rates were observed for hookworm infections [43].

In veterinary medicine, 4HR has demonstrated efficacy against a range of parasites in dogs [45]. However, some adverse effects have been noted, such as petechial hemorrhage in the stomach mucosa following oral administration [43]. Moreover, the use of 0.2% 4HR enemas for the removal of whipworms may lead to perianal skin irritation, necessitating precautions [23]. While there are alternative treatments available for parasitic infections, 4HR continues to be used in certain cases. It is essential to individualize the dosage and administration of 4HR based on the specific requirements and intended purpose of treatment. Further research is warranted to explore strategies to improve the oral bioavailability and minimize the potential adverse effects associated with the use of 4HR as an anthelmintic agent.

2.5 Hexylresorcinol in Lozenges

Airway infections commonly result from viral pathogens, which account for a significant majority, ranging from 85% to 95%, of adult sore throat cases [46]. In contrast, bacterial infections contribute to a relatively smaller proportion, typically around 5%–15% [47]. For the treatment of sore throat, lozenges containing 4HR have been utilized and have shown promising virucidal effects against parainfluenza virus type 3 and cytomegaloviruses [48]. Moreover, these lozenges have been observed to decrease viral titers by 85% and 91% for influenza A virus and human coronavirus OC43, respectively [49]. Interestingly, the independent form of 4HR exhibits similar antiviral efficacy to the 4HR-infused lozenges [48] (Fig. 2.6). The antiviral mechanism of action for 4HR is speculated to involve its interaction with viral lipid membranes or its modulation of protein-lipid interactions [50]. It is noteworthy to highlight that bacterial infections are rarely responsible for sore throat cases, constituting only a minority of 5%–15% [47].

4HR has been demonstrated to possess the ability to reversibly block depolarization-induced whole cell sodium inward currents, which offers potential for anesthetic effects when used in lozenges [51, 52]. In comparison to local anesthetics such as lidocaine, 4HR exhibits higher potency, being approximately 10–20 times more potent [51]. In cases of inflammatory tissue, the pain threshold is considerably lowered due to hypoxic damage and subsequent metabolic inhibition of the Na/K-ATPase [53]. The selectivity of 4HR in targeting depolarized nerve membranes enables its potential utilization in inhibiting high-frequency nerve discharges in damaged tissues [54]. The safety profile of 4HR has been evaluated in clinical studies. Specifically, in a study involving patients with sore throat, only one patient (2%) reported a mild adverse effect after receiving a 4HR lozenge containing 2.4 mg

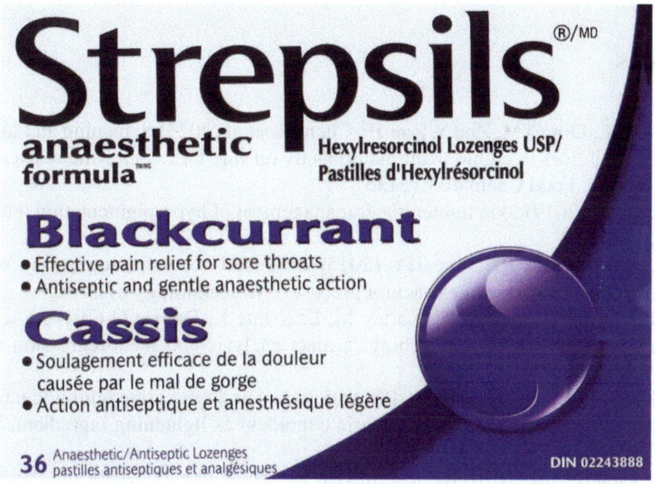

Fig. 2.6 Lozenges having 4HR as their ingredient

of the compound, while four patients (6%) in the placebo group reported mild adverse effects [52]. Therefore, the incidence of adverse effects with 4HR lozenges appears to be low.

Moreover, the therapeutic response to 4HR is prompt, with the analgesic effect observed within 1–5 min following oral administration, reaching its maximum at 15 min [52]. This rapid onset of action is noteworthy and may contribute to the clinical utility of 4HR in managing pain and inflammation in cases where a quick relief of symptoms is desired. Overall, the ability of 4HR to selectively target depolarized nerve membranes, its higher potency compared to lidocaine, and its favorable safety profile make it an interesting candidate for further exploration as an anesthetic agent, particularly in conditions characterized by inflammatory tissue and high-frequency nerve discharges. Further studies are warranted to fully elucidate its mechanism of action and evaluate its efficacy in different patient populations and clinical settings.

2.6 Closing Remark

The use of 4HR in cosmetics offers numerous advantages, and many commercial products containing this ingredient are readily available in the market. While 4HR is often used in lozenges due to its antiviral, antibacterial, and pain-relief properties, it is not particularly effective as an antiseptic, food additive, or anthelmintic compared to alternative substances. However, given its role as a histone deacetylase inhibitor, 4HR may hold promise for treating certain diseases and could potentially be used as an ingredient in nutraceuticals. Nonetheless, there is currently limited evidence available on this subject.

References

1. Fang X, Dai L, Ding TM, Zhu Y, Zan JF, Chen LL et al (2023) Screening and identification of tyrosinase inhibitors in edible plant materials by on-line UPLC-enzyme reactor coupled with UHPLC-FTMS. Food Chem 403:134331
2. Mohiuddin AK (2019) Skin lightening & management of hyperpigmentation. Pharma Sci Anal Res J 2(2):180020
3. Kim JS, Seo YC, No RH, Lee HY (2015) Improved cosmetic activity by optimizing the Lithospermum erythrorhizon extraction process. Cytotechnology 67:51–65
4. Sagoe D, Pallesen S, Dlova NC, Lartey M, Ezzedine K, Dadzie O (2019) The global prevalence and correlates of skin bleaching: a meta-analysis and meta-regression analysis. Int J Dermatol 58:24–44
5. Sari DM, Anwar E, Arifianti AE (2019) Antioxidant and tyrosinase inhibitor activities of ethanol extracts of brown seaweed (Turbinaria conoides) as lightening ingredient. Pharmacogn J 11:379–382
6. Arbab A, Eltahir MM (2010) Review on skin whitening agents. Khartoum Pharm J 13:5–9

7. Chiocchio I, Mandrone M, Sanna C, Maxia A, Tacchini M, Poli FJIC (2018) Screening of a hundred plant extracts as tyrosinase and elastase inhibitors, two enzymatic targets of cosmetic interest. Ind Crop Prod 122:498–505
8. Villareal MO, Kume S, Bourhim T, Bakhtaoui FZ, Kashiwagi K, Han J et al (2013) Activation of MITF by argan oil leads to the inhibition of the tyrosinase and dopachrome tautomerase expressions in B16 murine melanoma cells. Evid Based Complement Altern Med 2013:1–9
9. Michalek IM, Benn EK, Dos Santos FLC, Gordon S, Wen C, Liu B (2019) A systematic review of global legal regulations on the permissible level of heavy metals in cosmetics with particular emphasis on skin lightening products. Environ Res 170:187–193
10. Zhu W, Gao J (2008) The use of botanical extracts as topical skin-lightening agents for the improvement of skin pigmentation disorders. J Investig Dermatol Symp Proc 13:20–24
11. Mapunya MB, Hussein AA, Rodriguez B, Lall N (2011) Tyrosinase activity of Greyia flanaganii (bolus) constituents. Phytomedicine 18:1006–1012
12. Kozubek A, Tyman JH (1999) Resorcinolic lipids, the natural non-isoprenoid phenolic amphiphiles and their biological activity. Chem Rev 99:1–26
13. Makino ET, Mehta RC, Banga A, Jain P, Sigler ML, Sonti S (2013) Evaluation of a hydroquinone-free skin brightening product using in vitro inhibition of melanogenesis and clinical reduction of ultraviolet-induced hyperpigmentation. J Drugs Dermatol 12(3):s16–s20
14. Huber S, Mujica-Fernaud T (2009) Use of hydroxyphenylester-type tyrosinase inhibitors for skin lightening cosmetics. PCT Int Appl WO 2009021590. Chem Abstr 150:244611
15. Chaudhuri RK (2008) Skin lightening cosmetic compositions. U.S. pat Appl Publ US 20080305059. Chem Abstr 150:40863
16. Shariff R, Du Y, Dutta M, Kumar S, Thimmaiah S, Doraiswamy C et al (2022) Superior even skin tone and anti-ageing benefit of a combination of 4-hexylresorcinol and niacinamide. Int J Cosmet Sci 44(1):103–117
17. Fidalgo J, Deglesne PA, Arroya R, Ranneva E, Deprez P (2018) 4-hexylresorcinol a new molecule for cosmetic application. J Biomol Res Ther 8(1):170
18. Ortiz-Ruiz CV, Berna J, Rodriguez-Lopez JN, Tomas V, Garcia-Canovas F (2015) Tyrosinase-catalyzed hydroxylation of 4-hexylresorcinol, an antibrowning and depigmenting agent: a kinetic study. J Agric Food Chem 63(31):7032–7040
19. Hakozaki T, Minwalla L, Zhuang J, Chhoa M, Matsubara A, Miyamoto K et al (2002) The effect of niacinamide on reducing cutaneous pigmentation and suppression of melanosome transfer. Br J Dermatol 147(1):20–31
20. Wu H, Gabriel TA, Burney WA, Chambers CJ, Pan A, Sivamani RK (2023) Prospective, randomized, double-blind clinical study of split-body comparison of topical hydroquinone and hexylresorcinol for skin pigment appearance. Arch Dermatol Res 315(5):1207–1214
21. Draelos ZD, Diaz I, Cohen A, Mao J, Boyd T (2020) A novel skin brightening topical technology. J Cosmet Dermatol 19(12):3280–3285
22. Montero P, Martínez-Álvarez O, Zamorano JP, Alique R, Gómez-Guillén MC (2006) Melanosis inhibition and 4-hexylresorcinol residual levels in deepwater pink shrimp (Parapenaeus longirostris) following various treatments. Eur Food Res Technol 223:16–21
23. Jung RC, Beaver PC (1951) Clinical observations on Trichocepluflus trichuris (whip worm) infestation in children. Pediatrics 8:548
24. Sae-leaw T, Benjakul S, Simpson BK (2017) Effect of catechin and its derivatives on inhibition of polyphenoloxidase and melanosis of pacific white shrimp. J Food Sci Technol 54(5):1098–1107
25. Zolghadri S, Bahrami A, Hassan Khan MT, Munoz-Munoz J, Garcia-Molina F, Garcia-Canovas F et al (2019) A comprehensive review on tyrosinase inhibitors. J Enzyme Inhib Med Chem 34(1):279–309
26. Fang H, Tong W, Shi LM, Blair R, Perkins R, Branham W et al (2001) Structure-activity relationships for a large diverse set of natural, synthetic, and environmental estrogens. Chem Res Toxicol 14:280–294

27. Amadasi A, Mozzarelli A, Meda C, Maggi A, Cozzini P (2009) Identification of xenoestrogens in food additives by an integrated in silico and in vitro approach. Chem Res Toxicol 22(1):52–63
28. Hexylresorcinol, Compound summary, U.S. National Library of Medicine, NIH. https://pubchem.ncbi.nlm.nih.gov/ compound/ 3610#section = Metabolism-Metabolites. Accessed 17 Feb 2020
29. Shaffer A, Ramzy MM, Hegazy AI, Husseny AK, El-Hadary UG, Taha MM et al (2018) The molecular mechanisms of action of the endocrine disrupting chemical bisphenol a in the development of cancer. Gene 647:235–243
30. Hess-Wilson JK, Boldison J, Weaver KE, Knudsen KE (2006) Xenoestrogen action in breast cancer: impact on ER-dependent transcription and mitogenesis. Breast Cancer Res Treat 96(3):279–292
31. Lei B, Sun S, Zhang X, Feng C, Xu J, Wen Y et al (2019) Bisphenol AF exerts estrogenic activity in MCF-7 cells through activation of Erk and PI3K/Akt signals via GPER signaling pathway. Chemosphere 220:362–370
32. Kang YJ, Oh JH, Seok H, Jo YY, Kim DW, Garagiola U et al (2020) 4-hexylresorcinol exhibits different characteristics to estrogen. Appl Sci 10(5):1737
33. Newbold RR, Jefferson WN, Padilla-Banks E, Haseman J (2004) Developmental exposure to diethylstilbestrol (DES) alters uterine response to estrogens in prepubescent mice: low versus high dose effects. Reprod Toxicol 18(3):399–406
34. Ronchetti SA, Miler EA, Duvilanski BH, Cabilla JP (2013) Cadmium mimics estrogen-driven cell proliferation and prolactin secretion from anterior pituitary cells. PLoS One 8(11):e81101
35. Wilson CO, Gisvold O, Doerge RF (1971) Textbook of organic, medicinal, and pharmaceutical chemistry, 6th edn. J.B. Lippincott Co, Philadelphia, PA, pp 255–281
36. Feirer WA, Leonard V (1927) Hexylresorcinol in oral antisepsis with special reference to S.T. 37. D. Cosmos 64:882
37. Brown EA, Cruickshank GA (1947) A comparative study of the effects of glycerite of hydrogen peroxide and of hexylresorcinol on the bacteria of the normal mouth. J Dent Res 26(1):83–90
38. Twort CC, Baker AH (1942) Further researches on bactericidal mists and smokes. J Hyg (Lond) 42(3):266–283
39. Lidwell OM, Williams RE (1954) Trial of hexylresorcinol as air disinfectant for prevention of colds in office workers. Br Med J 2(4894):959–961
40. Evans RT, Baker PJ, Coburn RA, Fischman SL, Genco RJ (1977) In vitro antiplaque effects of antiseptic phenols. J Periodontol 48(3):156–162
41. Kraal JH, Hussain AA, Gregorio SB, Akaho E (1979) Exposure time and the effect of hexylresorcinol on bacterial aggregates. J Dent Res 58(11):2125–2131
42. Robinson HM Jr (1967) Effective antifungal drugs and indications for their use. Med Clin North Am 51(5):1181–1188
43. Maplestone PA, Mukerji AK (1932) Hexylresorcinol as an anthelmintic. Ind Med Gaz 67(11):610–612
44. Jung RC (1954) Use of a hexylresorcinol tablet in the enema treatment of whipworm infection. Am J Trop Med Hyg 3(5):918–921
45. Forbes LS (1964) The effect of certain substances against Echinococcus granulosus and Taenia hydatigena infections in dogs. Ann Trop Med Parasitol 58:132–146
46. Worrall G (2011) Acute sore throat. Can Fam Physician 57(7):791–794
47. Shulman ST, Bisno AL, Clegg HW, Gerber MA, Kaplan EL, Lee G et al (2012) Clinical practice guideline for the diagnosis and management of group a streptococcal pharyngitis: 2012 update by the Infectious Diseases Society of America. Clin Infect Dis 55(10):1279–1282
48. Shephard A, Zybeshari S (2015) Virucidal action of sore throat lozenges against respiratory viruses parainfluenza type 3 and cytomegalovirus. Antivir Res 123:158–162
49. Morokutti-Kurz M, Graf C, Prieschl-Grassauer E (2017) Amylmetacresol/2,4-dichlorobenzyl alcohol, hexylresorcinol, or carrageenan lozenges as active treatments for sore throat. Int J Gen Med 10:53–60

50. Oxford JS, Lambkin R, Gibb I, Balasingam S, Chan C, Catchpole A (2005) A throat lozenge containing amyl meta cresol and dichlorobenzyl alcohol has a direct virucidal effect on respiratory syncytial virus, influenza A and SARS-CoV. Antivir Chem Chemother 16(2):129–134
51. Buchholz V, Leuwer M, Ahrens J, Foadi N, Krampfl K, Haeseler G (2009) Topical antiseptics for the treatment of sore throat block voltage-gated neuronal sodium channels in a local anaesthetic-like manner. Naunyn Schmiedeberg's Arch Pharmacol 380(2):161–168
52. McNally D, Shephard A, Field E (2012) Randomised, double-blind, placebo-controlled study of a single dose of an amylmetacresol/2,4-dichlorobenzyl alcohol plus lidocaine lozenge or a hexylresorcinol lozenge for the treatment of acute sore throat due to upper respiratory tract infection. J Pharm Pharm Sci 15(2):281–294
53. Hammarstrom AK, Gage PW (1998) Inhibition of oxidative metabolism increases persistent sodium current in rat CA1 hippocampal neurons. J Physiol 510(Pt 3):735–741
54. Amir R, Argoff CE, Bennett GJ, Cummins TR, Durieux ME, Gerner P et al (2006) The role of sodium channels in chronic inflammatory and neuropathic pain. J Pain 7:S1–S29

Chapter 3
Anticancer Effects of 4-Hexylresorcinol

Abstract This chapter discusses the potential anti-tumor effect of 4-hexylresorcinol (4HR), a phenolic compound with antimicrobial and antioxidant properties. The chapter describes the biochemical properties of 4HR and its potential to suppress mitochondrial respiration, increase endoplasmic reticulum stress, and induce apoptosis in tumor cells. The chapter also details the results of in vitro and in vivo experiments with various cancer cell lines, demonstrating the efficacy of 4HR in reducing cancer cell proliferation. The chapter concludes by acknowledging the limitations of the study and the need for further research to confirm the anti-tumor effect of 4HR in other cancer cell lines and to determine its potential as an anticancer drug.

Keywords 4-hexylresorcinol (4HR) · Anti-tumor effect · Apoptosis · Cancer metabolism · Epithelial tumor

The anticancer properties of 4-hexylresorcinol (4HR) were first reported in the 1980s [1]. This discovery was made during a toxicology study, which suggested that 4HR and its derivatives may have potential as anticancer agents [2, 3]. In a national toxicological study, rats and mice were orally administered 4HR at dosages ranging from 31.3 to 500 mg/kg. The results showed that the administration of 4HR did not have any significant impact on animal survival, with no reported adverse effects observed, except for weight loss in healthy male rats receiving 250 or 500 mg/kg of 4HR [1]. When administered through subcutaneous injection, a dosage of 12.8 mg/kg of 4HR was found to cause a reduction in body weight in healthy growing male rats [4].

The findings of the study indicate that the incidence of spontaneous cancer is lower in the group treated with 4HR compared to the untreated control group. Specifically, the incidence of leukemia, hepatocellular carcinoma, and circulatory system tumors was reduced in the 4HR-treated group [1]. This could be attributed to the inhibitory effect of 4HR, a phenolic compound, on α-glycosidase and sorbitol dehydrogenase, which has been shown to be beneficial in the treatment of diabetes and leukemia [5]. In a xenograft study, the growth of implanted leukemia was also delayed with the administration of 4HR [6].

S.-G. Kim, *Biomedical Application of 4-Hexylresorcinol*,
https://doi.org/10.1007/978-981-97-0637-2_3

However, it is worth noting that some benign tumors showed an increased incidence in the male groups treated with 4HR. Specifically, the occurrence of pheochromocytoma in the adrenal and harderian gland was elevated [1]. It is important to consider that corn oil, used as a vehicle for 4HR in this study, may itself be inducing these tumors in mice [7]. Additionally, recent research has demonstrated that the size of the salivary gland is larger in the male group treated with 4HR compared to the untreated control group [8]. This could be attributed to the decrease in anabolic steroid levels, such as testosterone, with the administration of 4HR, leading to hyperplasia of glandular tissue as a compensatory response [8].

The compound 4HR is classified as a histone deacetylase inhibitor (HDACi), and as such, it is known to decrease the production of anabolic steroids such as testosterone in healthy growing animal models [4] through its inhibition of histone deacetylase enzymes. Consequently, the serum level of testosterone is reduced [4]. This reduction in testosterone levels has been linked to the observed decrease in body weight in male rats receiving 4HR [1, 4]. It is worth noting that the hyperplasia of the salivary gland, observed in response to 4HR administration, may be classified as reactive hyperplasia, potentially resulting from the decreased serum testosterone levels [8]. However, it is important to highlight that this reaction appears to be dependent on the systemic condition of the animals receiving the compound. For instance, in metabolically challenged models such as diabetes, the reactive hyperplasia in salivary glands is not observed. Diabetes associated effect is discussed in Chap. 8. The specific mechanisms underlying this difference need further investigation and are beyond the scope of this study. However, these findings suggest that the effects of 4HR administration, particularly the development of reactive hyperplasia, may vary based on the individual's systemic condition.

Cancer is abnormal situation. The metabolism in the cancer tissue is also different from the healthy tissue [9]. Cancer cells have loose cellular attachment. Therefore, their motility and migration to the adjacent structure are higher than those of normal cells [10]. When compared to microbiota, cancer cells mimic actively proliferating bacteria and are not looked like dormant bacteria. For the uncontrolled proliferation, the required energy is higher, and more glucose intake is needed [11]. Compared to mitochondrial respiration, aerobic glycolysis is low productivity in terms of ATP synthesis, but aerobic glycolysis is much more speedy process than mitochondrial respiration (Fig. 3.1). Considering the final amount of ATP in the limited time, aerobic glycolysis has a benefit for tumor cells compared to mitochondrial respiration. For the successful aerobic glycolysis, there are several conditions. First, cancer cells should win the competition in taking glucose against neighbor normal cells. Second, lactate dehydrogenase (LDH) should maintain its high activity to keep the aerobic glycolysis cycle. LDH is supplier of nicotinamide adenine dinucleotide+ (NAD+), and this is required for the activation of glyceraldehyde 3-phosphate dehydrogenase (GAPDH) (Fig. 3.2).

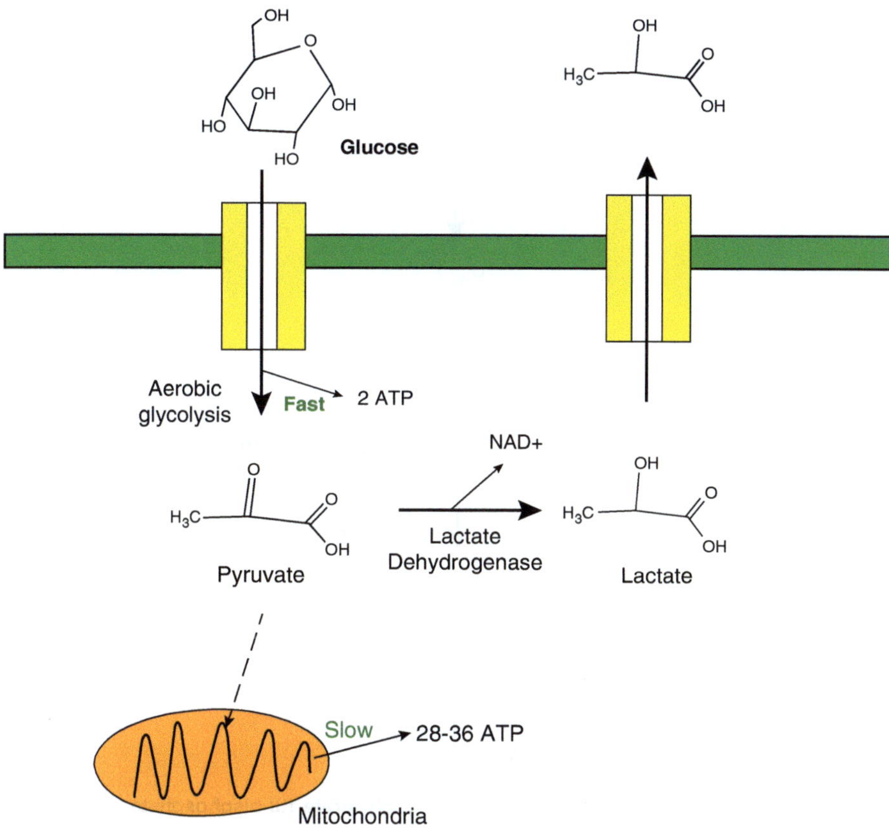

Fig. 3.1 Aerobic glycolysis produces two ATPs and one nicotinamide adenine dinucleotide+ (NAD+)

The effect of 4HR on the metabolic pathway in cancer cells remains unclear, although an unpublished result suggests that it may activate GAPDH. Further investigations are currently being conducted to elucidate the underlying mechanism. In the field of cancer research, several findings have been reported regarding the impact of 4HR on various pathways and proteins. It has been demonstrated that 4HR can inhibit the nuclear factor kappa B (NF-kB) pathway through the inhibition of transglutaminase-2 (TG-2) [12]. Additionally, 4HR has been shown to inhibit calcium oscillation [13]. Moreover, 4HR has been found to upregulate the expression of keratin and involucrin in carcinoma cells [14], both of which are known marker proteins for epithelial cell differentiation.

Furthermore, it has been observed that 4HR can bind to the DNA binding domain of mutant p53 and assist in its functional recovery [15]. Although these findings provide valuable insights into the potential effects of 4HR on various cellular processes, there is still a need for further research to fully understand the mechanisms

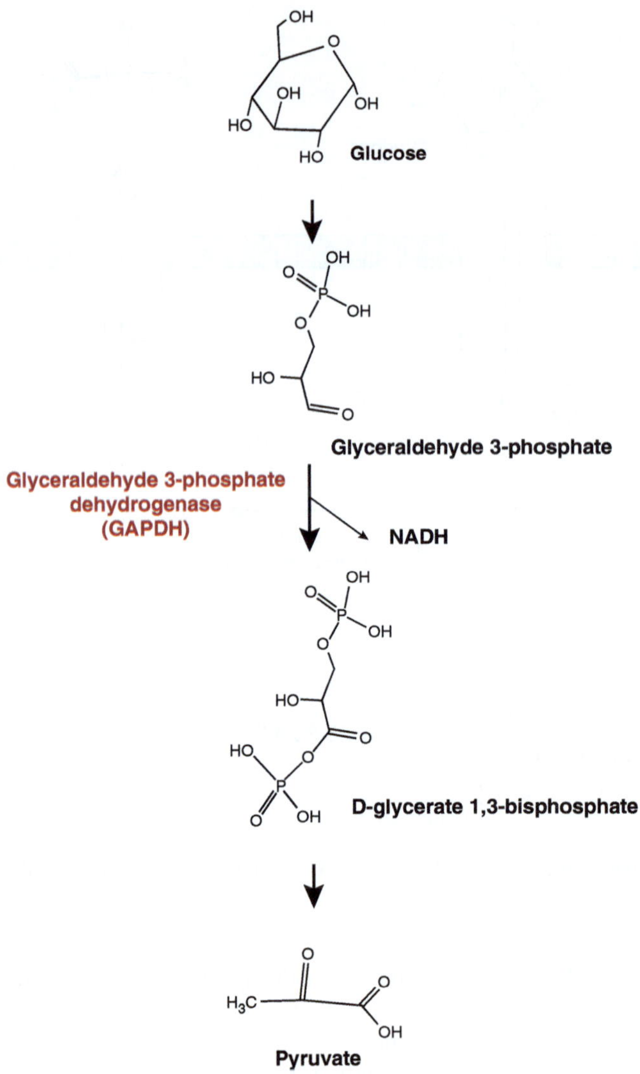

Fig. 3.2 Glyceraldehyde 3-phosphate dehydrogenase (GAPDH) is required to produce pyruvate. For the activation of GAPDH, NAD+ is required. NAD+ is reduced to NADH and makes D-glyerate 1,3-bisphosphate

underlying these observations. It is crucial to determine if 4HR truly alters the metabolic pathway in cancer cells and how this relates to its effects on GAPDH activation. Therefore, ongoing investigations will contribute to a more comprehensive understanding of the impact of 4HR on cancer cells and may open new avenues for therapeutic interventions in the future. Until then, caution should be exercised in interpreting these preliminary findings.

3.1 NF-κB Pathway Inhibition

NF-κB is a transcription factor, and its signaling pathway is involved in various cellular events [16]. The target genes for NF-κB are involved in inflammation, angiogenesis, and cellular proliferation [17, 18]. Accordingly, the abnormal activation of NF-κB pathway is frequently found in tumors [16]. The inhibition of NF-κB pathway can increase the apoptosis of tumor cells [19]. Accordingly, NF-κB pathway is considered as a therapeutic target of tumor.

In resting state, NF-κB is bound to the nuclear factor of kappa light polypeptide gene enhancer in B-cell inhibitor (IκB) [21]. When activation signal is transmitted through receptor, NF-κB is phosphorylated and dissociated from IκB (Fig. 3.3). Phosphorylated NF-κB is translocated into the nucleus. Phosphorylated NF-κB in the nucleus behaves like transcription factor [22]. When free NF-κB is transported to the cytoplasm again, it can be stabilized via binding to IκB. TG-2 is a glue-like protein and involved in IκB polymerization [23]. When TG-2 is activated, free NF-κB will be increased by IκB polymerization [23]. This activation is associated with the resistance against chemotherapy [24].

Though TG-2 is mainly found in the cytoplasm, it can be found elsewhere such as nucleus and mitochondria [25]. Intra-nuclear localization can be interpreted as high level of TG-2 activity [26]. The cancer cells showing abnormal activation of NF-κB pathway also exhibit intra-nuclear localization of TG-2 [20]. As TG-2 is found with the p65 subunit of NF-kB in the cytoplasm, translocation of p65 will increase TG-2 translocation, too [24]. When 4HR is administered to these cancer cells, the level of TG-2 nuclear localization is decreased (Fig. 3.4).

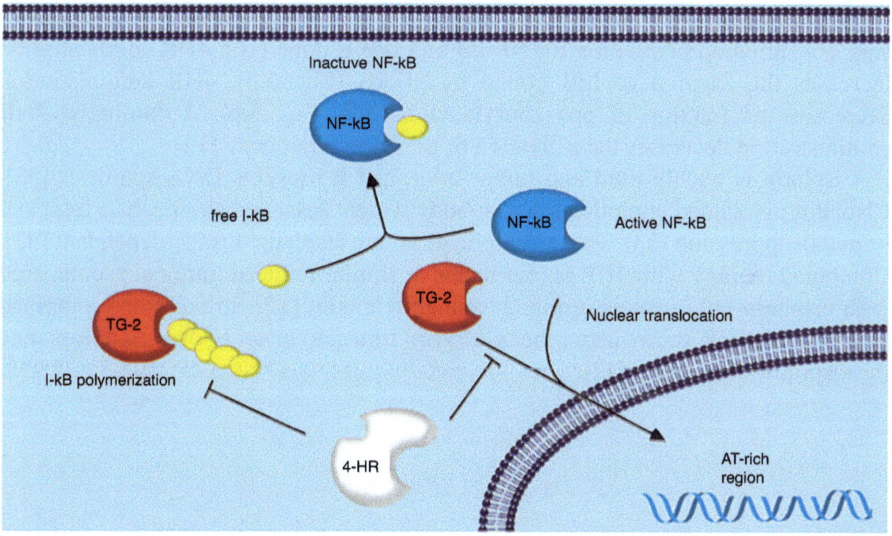

Fig. 3.3 Schematic drawing for the role of TG-2 and the effect of 4HR administration (reproduced from author's own publication [20])

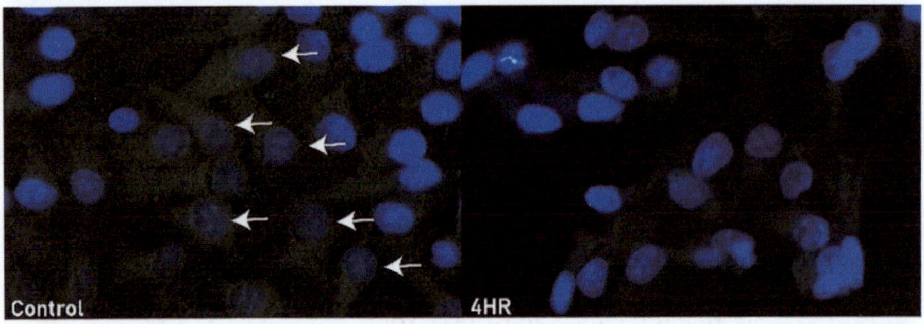

Fig. 3.4 Nasopharyngeal cancer cell line (KB cell) is stained by FITC-conjugated TG-2 antibody and 4′,6-diamidino-2-phenylindole (DAPI). Untreated control shows intra-nuclear localization of TG-2 (arrows). However, 4HR treatment decreases intra-nuclear localization of TG-2 as shown DAPI signal only in the nucleus (Modified from author' own publication [20])

The administration of NF-kB inhibitor decreases and blocks TG-2 expression and NF-kB nuclear translocation [27]. Translocated NF-kB binds to AT-rich regions of the target genes [28]. 4′,6-Diamidino-2-phenylindole (DAPI) binds to similar area, too [29]. If 4HR inhibits NF-kB nuclear translocation, AT-rich regions of the target genes will be vacant and can be used for DAPI binding. Compared to the untreated control group, 4HR administration increases the fluorescence lifetime of DAPI (Fig. 3.5). The elongated average lifetime in 4HR group is caused by a tightly bound DAPI-DNA complex, which is a long lifetime component [30, 31]. If NF-kB cannot translocate into the nucleus, free AT-rich regions in the nucleus may be available for DAPI binding (Fig. 3.5).

When cell receives NF-κB activation signal, IκB proteins bound to NF-κB will be degraded [22]. To analyze the effect of 4HR administration on the NF-κB pathway, co-immunoprecipitation for NF-κB and IκB is done [12]. 4HR administration increases the fraction of IκB bound to NF-κB (Fig. 3.6). 4HR administration decreases the fraction of phosphorylated NF-κB (Fig. 3.6). Accordingly, 4HR administration decreases the activation of the NF-κB pathway [12].

Cisplatin is widely used anti-tumor drug, and it prevents DNA synthesis [32]. Cisplatin-associated complications are body weight loss, xerostomia, hair loss, and immunosuppression [33]. These complications are cisplatin dosage-dependent [33]. Combined therapy with 4HR shows better or similar reduced tumor size compared with cisplatin-only groups in tumor xenograft model [12]. In addition, combined therapy with 4HR shows better mean survival time and lower body weight loss than the cisplatin-only group [12].

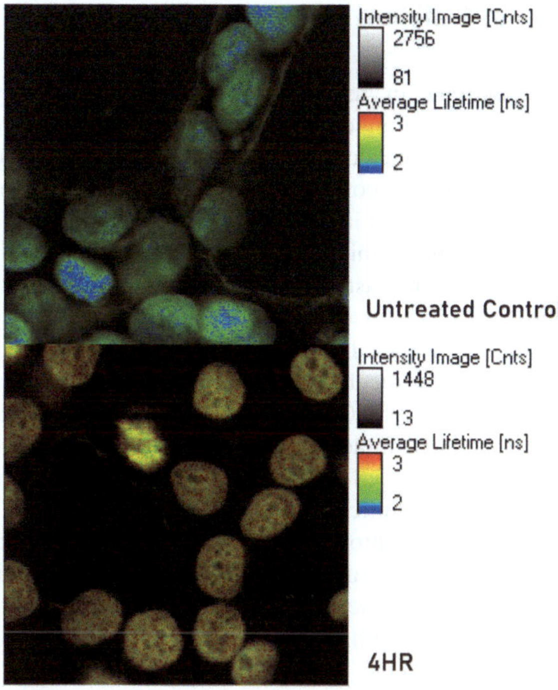

Fig. 3.5 Lifetime confocal images. Untreated control group shows intense blue spectrum in the nucleus attributed to short lifetime. In contrary to untreated control, 4HR treatment group shows yellow-to-red spectrum in the nucleus attributed to long lifetime (Modified from author' own publication [20])

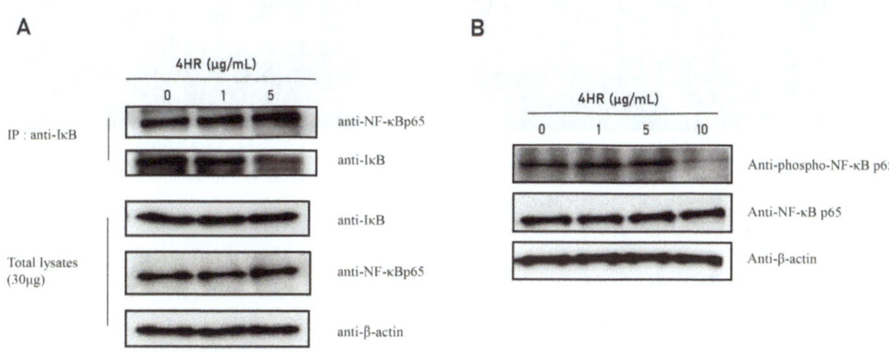

Fig. 3.6 Western blot (WB) for the evaluation of 4HR administration on KB cells. (**a**) Co-immunoprecipitation for NF-κB and IκB. Free IκB is decreased by 4HR administration. (**b**) Phosphorylated NF-κB fraction is decreased by 4HR administration (Modified from author' own publication [12])

3.2 Inhibition of Calcium Oscillation

Calcium ion is important in regulating cellular differentiation and growth. Particularly, intracellular calcium ion should be upregulated for the cellular apoptosis. The change of intracellular calcium concentration can be tracked by fluorescent calcium tracker using live cell confocal microscopy [13]. As shown in Fig. 3.7, intracellular calcium is increased in SCC-9 cells by 4HR administration compared with control cells. Interestingly, this calcium increase by 4HR administration is not evident in normal dermal fibroblasts. However, calcium oscillation is suppressed in both types of cells (Fig. 3.7).

Caspase-3/7 is a key caspase for the induction of cellular apoptosis. For the activation of caspase-3/7, intracellular calcium ion concentration should be elevated. 4HR administration on SCC-9 cells increases the appearance of apoptotic bodies on their surface [13]. In addition, the activity of caspase-3/7 is elevated by 4HR administration (Fig. 3.8). If elevated level of intracellular calcium is required for 4HR-mediated anticancer effect, calcium blockers may attenuate 4HR-mediated cancer cell apoptosis. Amlodipine and diltiazem are well-known calcium channel blockers. Treatment of either amlodipine or diltiazem before 4HR administration attenuates 4HR-mediated caspase-3/7 activation. Consequently, 4HR-mediated inhibition on cancer cell growth is also attenuated by calcium channel blocker [13].

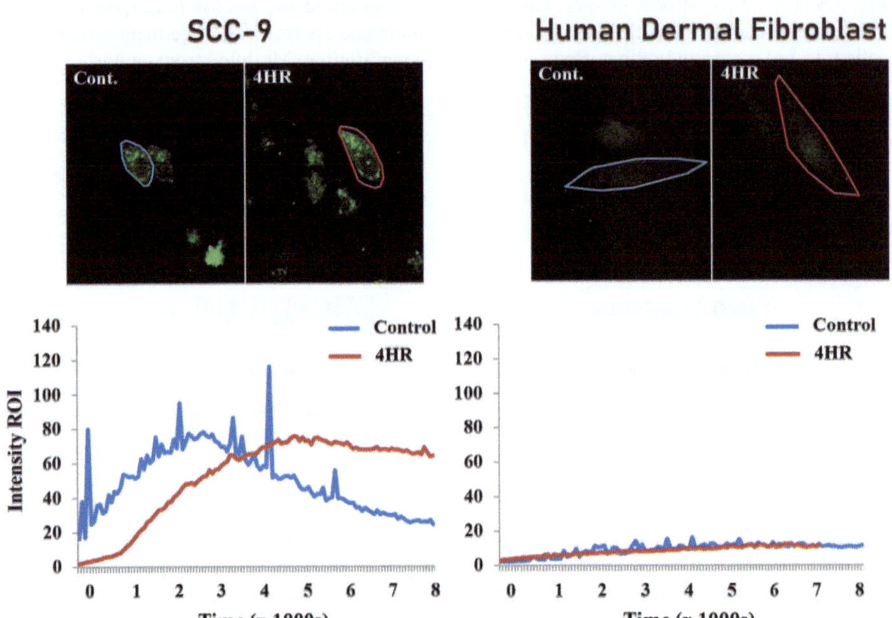

Fig. 3.7 Intracellular calcium tracking. 4HR treatment (10 μg/mL) inhibits calcium oscillation and maintains calcium concentration as high level in both the tongue cancer cell (SCC-9) and normal human dermal fibroblast (Modified from author' own publication [13])

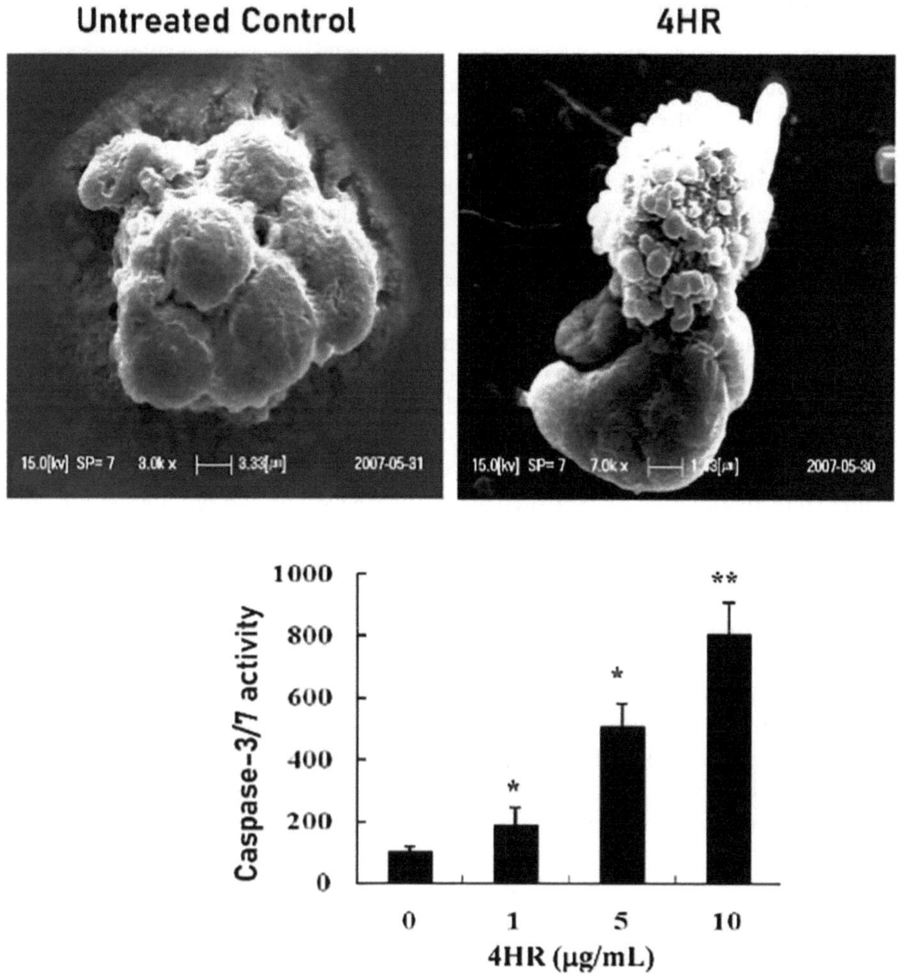

Fig. 3.8 Scanning electron microscopic (SEM) image and caspase-3/7 assay. Multiple apoptotic bodies are observed on the surface of cancer cells in 4HR group. The administration of 4HR increases the activity of caspase-3/7 in SCC-9 cells in a dose-dependent manner (*$P < 0.05$, **$P < 0.005$) (Modified from author' own publication [13])

Intracellular calcium introduction is mediated by voltage-dependent calcium channels [34]. The different level of calcium introduction between SCC-9 cells and normal dermal human fibroblasts may be due to the difference in the distribution of glutamate receptor. Glutamate receptor is responsible for calcium oscillation [35, 36]. In addition, the expression level of glutamate receptor in oral squamous cell carcinoma is much higher than that in normal oral epithelium [37]. Accordingly, 4HR-mediated inhibition of calcium oscillation will have much more impact on tumors than normal tissue. The administration of glutamate receptor inhibitor inhibits cancer cell growth, but not in normal dermal fibroblast [38].

3.3 Differentiation of Carcinoma

As tumor cells proliferate in uncontrolled manner, the signaling pathways associated with cellular differentiation and senescence are in the state of silence. The way of revertant is unclear in case of tumor cells. However, tumor differentiation therapy has been tried for decades [39]. Excluding some types of congenital tumours, most tumor cells are transformed normal cells due to carcinogenic stimuli. Several key genes responsible for cellular senescence are mutated, and their function is lost in tumors [40]. The purpose of tumor differentiation therapy is a recovery of differentiation machinery by bypassing the mutated pathway.

E2F is a transcription factor and often highly expressed in tumors [41]. The aberrant activity of E2F is associated with uncontrolled growth and dedifferentiation in the carcinoma [42]. The genes transcribed by E2F are related to DNA synthesis and cell cycle progression [43, 44]. When the activity of E2F is inhibited, cellular proliferation is decreased [45]. Additionally, E2F inhibition increases the expression of epithelial differentiation marker such as involucrin [39]. In our previous study [14], the administration of 4HR to SCC-9 cells decreases the expression level of E2F2 and E2F3 (Fig. 3.9). In addition, involucrin and keratin 10 are increased by 4HR administration (Fig. 3.10). Ki67 is a marker for cellular proliferation. In xenograft model, 4HR administration results in decrease of Ki67 expression level, but increase of keratin 10 [14]. Therefore, 4HR administration decreases the expression level of E2F2, E2F3, and Ki67 but increases the expression level of epithelial differentiation markers such as involucrin and keratin 10 (Figs. 3.9 and 3.10).

Cellular senescence is defined as a cellular aging process without permanent activation of cell cycle [46]. Therefore, inactivation of cell cycle and restoring cellular differentiation program would be invaluable for tumor treatment [39]. For the

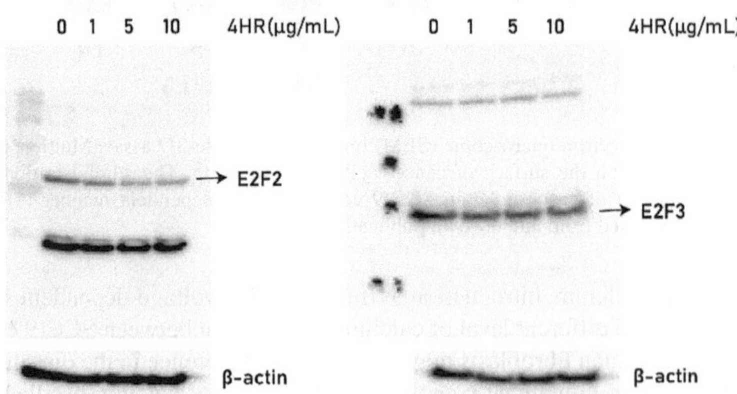

Fig. 3.9 The expression level of E2F2 and E2F3 after 4HR administration in SCC-9 cells. 4HR administration decreases the expression level of E2F2 and E2F3 in SCC-9 cells (Full-length Western blot used for author's previous publication [14])

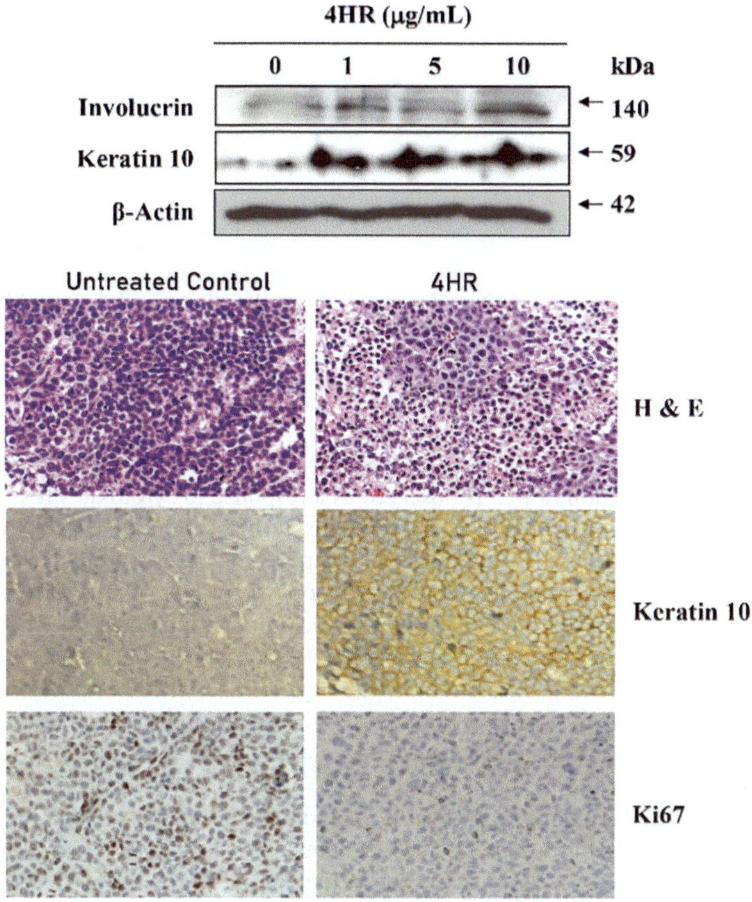

Fig. 3.10 The expression level of involucrin and keratin 10 after 4HR administration in SCC-9 cells. 4HR administration increases the expression level of involucrin and keratin 10 in SCC-9 cells. This trend is also observed in the immunohistochemical analysis of tissue specimen from tumor xenograft model (Modified from author' own publication [14])

successful differentiation therapy, the suppression of E2F signaling pathway is important step. The differentiation of epithelial tumor is regulated by Sp1 and E2F [47]. When Sp1 is increased, the cellular differentiation is activated and E2F is a negative regulator [39]. When E2F1, E2F2, and E2F3 are highly expressed, cellular differentiation is suppressed [48]. For the successful differentiation therapy, both E2F and Sp1 should be controlled [39]. The administration of 4HR increases the expression level of Sp1, too [14].

E2F suppression is a key element of keratinocyte differentiation [41]. E2F suppression by 4HR administration is important in 4HR-induced differentiation therapy (Fig. 3.11).

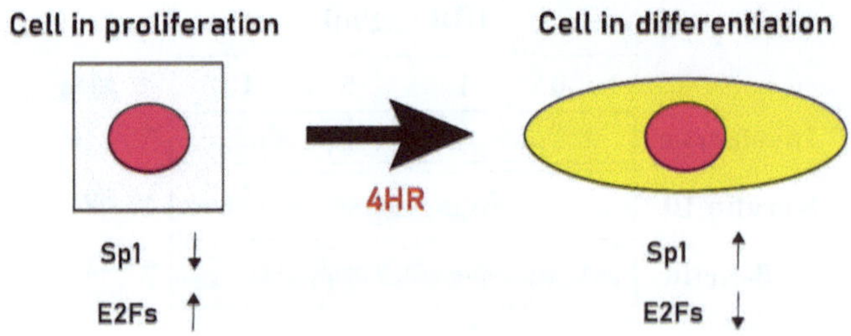

Fig. 3.11 The proposed mechanism of tumor cell differentiation by 4HR administration. The administration of 4HR increases expression level of Sp1 but decreases expression level of E2Fs

3.4 Functional Recovery of TP53

The mutation of TP53 is a frequent finding of carcinoma in the head and neck area [49, 50]. The activation of p53 is observed as a response to cytotoxic stress such as DNA damage [51]. Activated p53 is a tetramer with acetylation and phosphorylation [52]. After translocation into the nucleus, p53 binds to the promoter of genes, which transcribes genes associated with the apoptosis or DNA damage repair [51]. TP53 is a gene for p53 [53]. If TP53 shows concomitant mutation with other genes, mutant p53 cannot trigger cellular apoptosis [54]. Consequently, tumor cells can go to uncontrolled cellular proliferation despite high levels of TP53 or p53 expression [55]. Some types of mutant p53 can act as gain-of-function [50, 56]. In this case, tumor invasion and angiogenesis can be accelerated with the help of mutant p53 [50, 56].

Inactivated and mutant p53 is not able to bind to the promoter region of the genes associated with cellular apoptosis [54]. Mutant p53 can interact with other transcription factors that are responsible for invasive tumor growth [56]. Most mutations in TP53 are found in the promoter-binding area [57]. YD-15 is a mucoepidermoid carcinoma cell line in the oral cavity that has a mutation in TP53 [58]. YD-15 has an amino acid change mutation from aspartic acid (hydrophilic) to alanine (hydrophobic) in the DNA-binding domain [58]. This amino acid change influences the DNA-binding ability of p53. Protein conformation change will influence its phosphorylation and acetylation because of potential hiding of the activation domain. Consequently, YD-15 does not undergo apoptosis despite a high level of p53 expression (Fig. 3.12).

The treatment strategy for carcinoma that has a mutation in TP53 is restoring p53 function [59]. The strategy can be classified into the following three categories: (1) targeting degradation or direct inhibition of mutant p53; (2) binding to mutant p53 and inducing conformation change to a desirable form; and (3) targeting the viral enzymes that are responsible for the degradation of p53 [59]. Small molecules that can bind to mutant p53, inducing mutant p53 conformation change, have been a specific focus in recent studies [59]. PRIMA-1, APR-246, and CP-31398 are the chemicals that can bind to p53, inducing mutant p53 conformation change [59]. Though these chemicals are interesting in terms of restoring mutant p53 conformation, they generate reactive oxygen species (ROS) via suppressing antioxidant

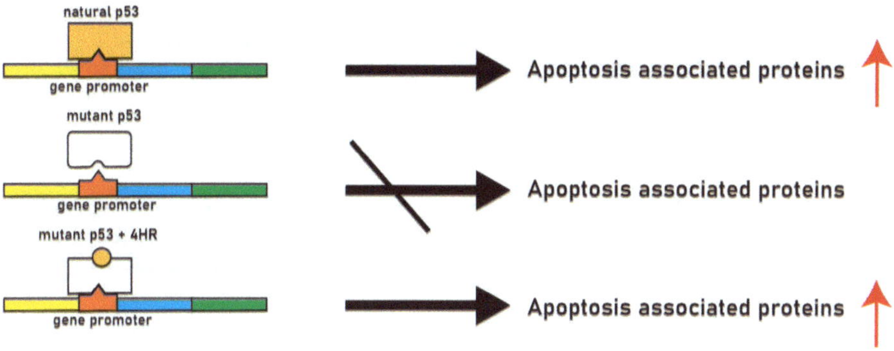

Fig. 3.12 The proposed mechanism of mutant p53 reactivation by 4HR administration. As mutant p53 has a mutation in its DNA-binding domain, mutant p53 can be expected to have less transcription activity. When 4HR is coupled with mutant p53, its DNA-binding activity may be increased by its conformation change. Consequently, p53 transcription activity will be recovered (reproduced from author's previous publication [15])

enzymes [60]. Though ROS may provide additional toxicity to cancer cells, ROS is also carcinogenic and toxic to normal cells [61]. This is a limitation for the clinical application of these chemicals [60]. Therefore, chemicals that can change mutant p53 conformation and have antioxidant properties should be investigated. Additionally, the inhibition of histone deacetylase (HDAC) can increase the level of acetylation of p53 and assist with its the activation [62, 63].

4HR is a pharmacologic chaperone that has antioxidant properties [64, 65] and is an HDAC inhibitor [66]. The administration of 4HR induces endoplasmic reticulum (ER)-mediated stress potentially by protein folding changes [64]. When 4HR is administered to human umbilical vein endothelial cells (HUVECs), the expression level of transforming growth factor-β1 (TGF-β1) increased [67]. This is a combined action of ER stress and HDAC inhibition [64]. When 4HR is provided to microorganisms under heating/radiation, the macromolecules in the cell are stabilized by 4HR [68]. Collectively, 4HR may recover p53 DNA-binding activity via its binding to mutant p53 and conformation change of mutant p53. This conformation change may recover the function of mutant p53. In addition, HDAC inhibition by 4HR can increase the acetylation of p53 [69], and this will help the activation of p53. Consequently, tumor cell may undergo cellular apoptosis by the action of recovered p53.

4HR administration increased the acetylation and phosphorylation of p53 in YD-15 cells (Fig. 3.13). The expression level of HDAC4 was decreased by 4HR administration [69]. YD-15 cells had a p53 mutation in its DNA-binding domain [58]. When 4HR is applied to the mutant peptide, its conformation was changed and close to that of normal p53 [15]. The administration of 4HR increases p53 transcription activity in both YD-9 and YD-15 cells [15]. The expression level of Bcl-2-associated death promoter (Bad) and Bcl-2-associated X protein (Bax) is increased by p53 administration in both YD-9 and YD-15 cells [15]. The apoptosis induced by 4HR is confirmed by cytochrome c leakage in YD-15 cells after 4HR administration [15].

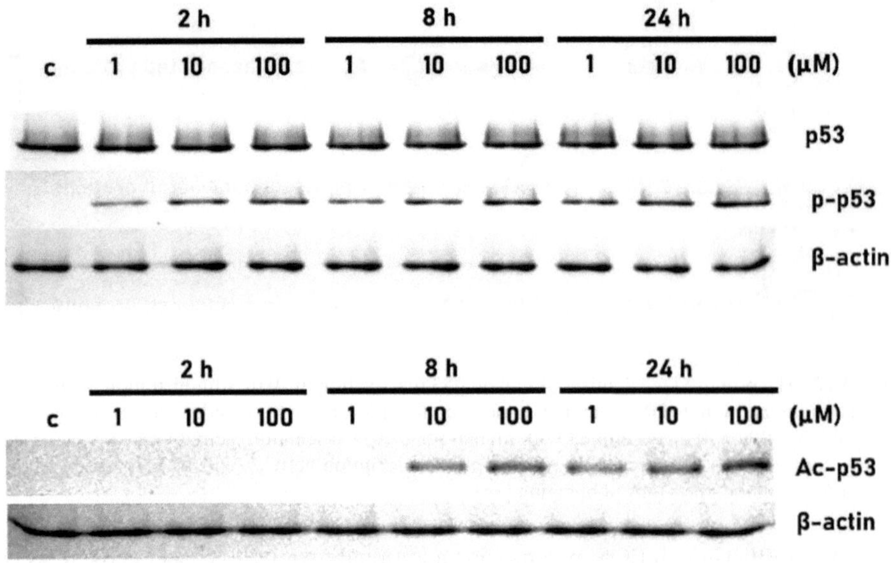

Fig. 3.13 The change of p53 expression level by 4HR administration in YD15 cell. The administration of 4HR does not change p53 expression level but increases the expression level of phosphorylated p53 (p-p53) and acetylated p53 (Ac-p53) (modified from author's previous publication [69])

TP53 mutation is a frequent finding in oral cancer [49, 50]. Several strategies against mutant TP53 have been developed [50]. The most frequent site of TP53 mutation is the DNA-binding site [51]. Mutant p53 may not bind properly to DNA, and its transcription activity will be lowered compared to normal p53 [51]. Consequently, the expression level of genes associated with apoptosis is lowered, and their protein expression level is also decreased [50, 51]. Glutamic acid at the 258th amino acid in p53 was replaced by alanine in YD-15 cells [58]. The peptide around the mutant site is designed and synthesized (Fig. 3.14). The conformation of the peptide from mutant p53 is predicted to have a random coil structure, but the conformation of peptide from normal p53 was a β-sheet structure [15]. Interestingly, the administration of p53 changed the conformation of the peptide from mutant p53 and brought it close to that of the peptide from normal p53 (Fig. 3.14). This conformation change of mutant p53 by 4HR administration should improve the transcription activity of p53. The transcription activity of p53 is significantly increased by 4HR administration in both YD-15 and YD-9 cells [15]. Several chemicals have been identified that could change the conformation of mutant p53 [59]. However, most of these increase the production of reactive oxygen species (ROS) [59]. Therefore, while they may be helpful for killing tumor cells, they will also induce toxicity in normal organs by its systemic administration [70]. Compared to previous conformation change chemicals, 4HR has antioxidant activity [71, 72]. Thus, its systemic application would be relatively safe compared to others [72].

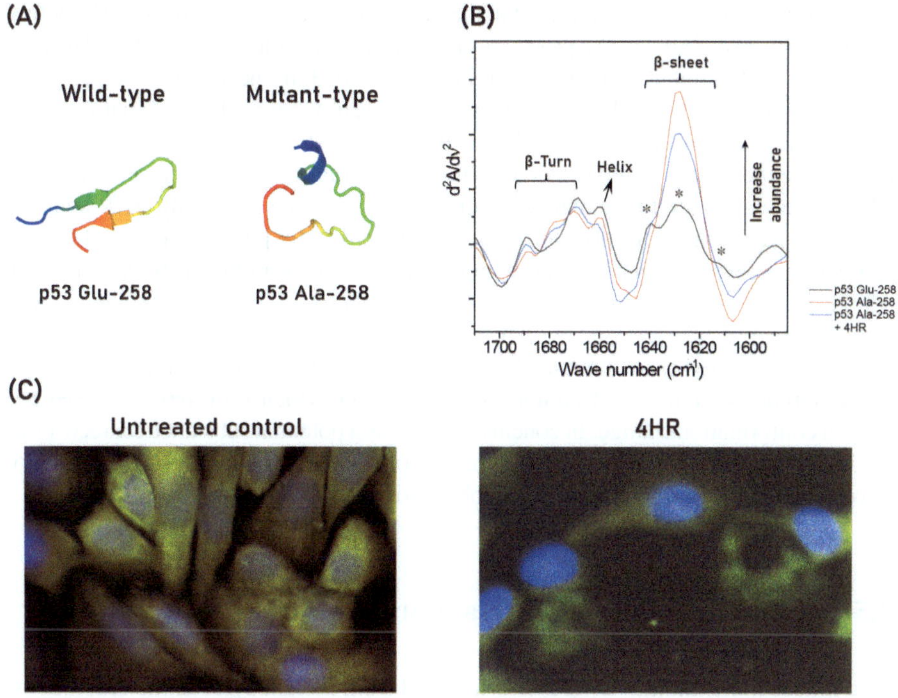

Fig. 3.14 The change of p53 conformation by 4HR administration. (**a**) Peptides are synthesized in the mutant area of p53. Glutamic acid at the 258th amino acid in p53 was replaced by alanine in YD-15 cells. Predicted structure is different between wild type and mutant type. (**b**) Using synthesized peptides, actual peptide structure is studied using Fourier transform infrared spectroscopy. Actual peptide structure is in accord to the prediction. Interestingly, 4HR administration on mutant type (blue) changes its conformation close to wild type (red). (**c**) 4HR administration increases cytochrome c release from the mitochondria (modified from author's previous publication [15])

The transcription factor is activated by acetylation and phosphorylation [73]. Accordingly, p53 activation and its transportation into the nucleus are achieved by p53 acetylation and phosphorylation [74]. As HDAC removes the acetyl group from the target protein, its inhibitor increases the acetylation of target protein [62]. 4HR is a Class I HDAC inhibitor [66]. The administration of 4HR increases the acetylation level of p53 in both YD-9 and YD-15 cells [69]. Phosphorylation is also important for signal transduction [75]. The administration of 4HR also increased the phosphorylation of p53 in both YD-9 and YD-15 cells [69]. Increased transcription activity of p53 in YD-9 and YD-15 cells is believed to be due to p53 activation and conformation change (Fig. 3.14). The administration of 4HR increases the expression level of TP53 and Bad mRNA, significantly ($p < 0.001$) [69].

The administration of 4HR in the xenograft model shows an improved survival rate [69] and reduced tumor mass [15]. As the ectopic tumor formation rate of YD-15 cell is notoriously low [58], both studies [15, 69] have low sample number. The tumorigenicity of YD-15 cells is 0/5 in athymic nude mouse [58]. Despite this limitation, the expression level of p-p53 and Ac-p53 is elevated in the 4HR administration group [69]. The activation of p53 is also found in the protein array analysis of the blood serum [69]. The level of murine double minute 2 (Mdm2), an inhibitor of p53, in the serum is decreased by 4HR administration [69]. The expression level of serum extracellular signal-regulated kinase 8 (ERK8) has been decreased in aggressive breast and lung cancers [76]. ERK8 inhibits the motility of tumor cells [76]. The administration of 4HR increases the serum ERK8 level compared to the untreated control [76]. In a previous study, 4HR administration decreased the metastasis of tumor cells, significantly [20]. The elevated level of serum caspase 9 and signal transducer and activator of transcription 4 (STAT4) by 4HR administration may be associated with p53 activation [69]. The phosphorylation levels of p53 at Ser315 are increased by 4HR administration, but those at Ser9 and Ser46 are decreased compared to the untreated control [69]. The change in phosphorylation level at a different location in p53 protein may be indirect evidence of 4HR-mediated p53 protein conformation change. In conclusion, 4HR is a potential substance for recovering the loss-of-function in mutant p53 as a pharmacologic chaperone and via the acetylation of p53 with HDAC4 inhibition and p53 phosphorylation.

3.5 Inhibition of Matrix Metalloproteinases

Oral mucosal melanoma (OMM) is originated from melanocytes in the oral mucosa and mostly found in the palate [77]. OMM shows aggressive infiltrative growth poor prognosis [78]. OMM responds poorly to chemotherapy/radiotherapy [79] and surgical excision with safe margin is recommended [80]. Considering its aggressive infiltrative growth through the lymphatic and vascular systems, early regional metastasis is common [77]. Regional lymph node metastasis is found in 25–50% of OMM patients at the time of diagnosis [78]. Distant OMM metastases are also frequently observed in the skin, lung, and brain [81]. In case of incomplete resection, it is possible for malignant cells to disseminate after surgical resection [77].

Several drugs, including cisplatin, cisplatin plus 4HR, deticene, tamoxifen, and imatinib, are applied to cultured primary OMM cells for preliminary evaluation of their anticancer effects (Fig. 3.15). Deticene [83], tamoxifen [84], and imatinib [85] have been used for the treatment of melanoma. However, they are mainly used for skin malignant melanoma and few data for OMM. As there can be many variations in OMM, primary cultured OMM cell from a patient may have limited information. Considering limitation of study, presented OMM cells are most effectively inhibited by cisplatin plus 4HR administration (Fig. 3.15).

4HR inhibits transglutaminase-2 and the NF-κB pathway in OSCC [12, 20], which controls the expression of many growth factors, including matrix metalloproteinases (MMPs) [86]. The expression level of MMP-2 is also regulated by TGF-β1 in oral squamous cell carcinoma [87]. The administration of 4HR can increase the expression level of TGF-β1 [67]. If the expression of MMPs in OMM is dependent on NF-κB pathway, the administration of 4HR will be beneficial for the treatment of OMM. If the expression of MMPs in OMM is dependent on TGF-β1, the

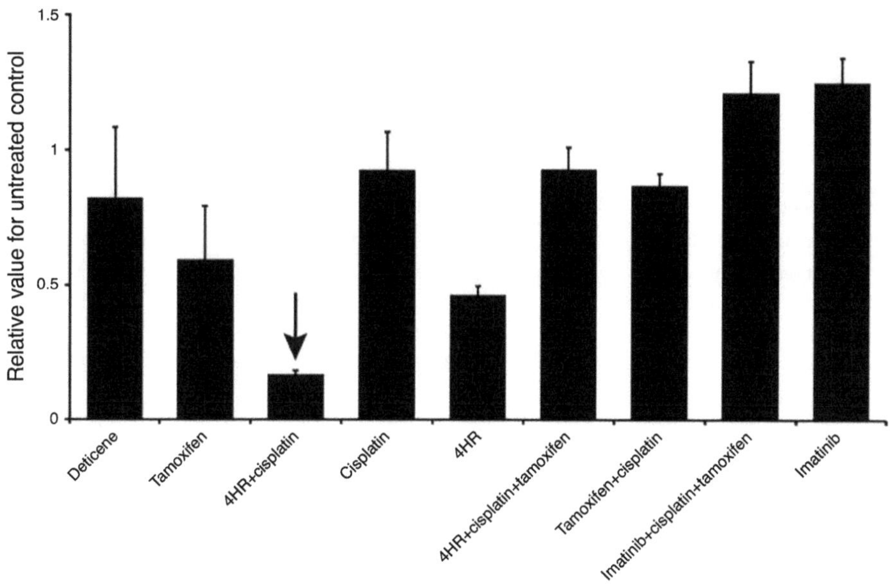

Fig. 3.15 Nine different combinations of chemotherapeutic agents are tested on primary cultured OMM cells. Untreated control value is set as 1. Some combinations show more than 1. Among these combination, 4HR + cisplatin combination (arrow) shows best result (modified from author's previous publication [82])

administration of 4HR will be a disaster for the treatment of OMM. In our cDNA microarray analysis, the expression levels of MMP−1, −2, and − 3 were low, while that of TIMP-2 was high after the application of 10 μg/mL of 4HR (Table 3.1). Microarray results are confirmed by subsequent quantitative reverse transcriptase-polymerase chain reaction and Western blot for selected targets (Fig. 3.16).

Several candidate agents have been tested as treatments for OMM, but the results are not promising [88]. Combination therapy with immunologic agents for OMM has been reported, too [89]. The outcome of combination therapy is 21.8% for the 5-year cumulative survival rate and 65.7% for distant metastasis [77]. Melanin is produced by tyrosinase [90], and 4HR can inhibit tyrosinase activity [91]. If melanin synthesis is important in OMM progression, its inhibition may have therapeutic advantage. However, some OMMs are amelanotic [92, 93]. As shown in Fig. 3.17, primary lesion in the palate and metastatic lesion of OMM were pigmented. Implanted OMM cells in the animal model did not have any pigmentation [82]. However, the metastatic tumor cells in the lung and the kidney of the experimental animals were melanotic [82]. Considering the interchanging amelanotic and melanotic phenotypes of OMM cells, melanin production may not be the optimal target pathway for therapy.

In our xenograft studies, (1) 2.5 mg/kg of cisplatin and (2) 1.25 mg/kg of cisplatin plus 2.5 mg/kg of 4HR were administered daily by intraperitoneal injection [82]. 4HR is usually administered orally, but few fractions are absorbed systemically in case of oral administration. To achieve therapeutic level of 4HR for OMM treatment, 4HR

Table 3.1 cDNA microarray results for primary cultured oral malignant melanoma cells after 4HR administration (modified from author's previous publication [82])

Title	Genbank	Chromosome	Fold-ratio
Tyrosine kinase 2	NM_003331	19p13.2	−4.187
Melanoma antigen family D, 2	NM_201222	Xp11.2	−3.438
Melanophilin	NM_024101	2q37.3	−19.971
Melanoregulin	NM_018000	2q35	−2.686
Matrix metallopeptidase 1	NM_002421	11q22.3	−11.509
Matrix metallopeptidase 2	BQ010172	16q13-q21	−6.300
Matrix metallopeptidase 3	NM_002422	11q22.3	−7.465
Interleukin 8	NM_000584	4q13-q21	−2.265
Interleukin 3	NM_000588	5q31.1	−2.628
Bone morphogenetic protein 1	NM_006128	8p21.3	−5.468
Bone morphogenetic protein 4	NM_001202	14q22-q23	−2.009
Bone morphogenetic protein 6	NM_001718	6p24-p23	−4.430
TIMP metallopeptidase inhibitor 2	NM_003255	17q25	3.394
Interferon, gamma	NM_000619	12q14	4.237

should be administered via parenteral route. The median lethal doses of 4HR in mice were 50 mg/kg and 750 mg/kg when injected intraperitoneally and subcutaneously, respectively [1]. Cisplatin is widely used as an anticancer drug. A single intraperitoneal injection of at least 7.5 mg/kg of cisplatin inhibited tumor growth significantly in a human squamous cell carcinoma xenograft model [94]. In our study, given the rapid disease progression of the OMM, we administered more doses of cisplatin than in other studies [94, 95]. 4HR and cisplatin combination group shows significantly lower MMP-2 expression than cisplatin-only group ($p < 0.001$) [82]. In addition, 4HR and cisplatin combination group shows significantly fewer distant metastases and a longer survival period than the cisplatin-only group ($p < 0.05$) [82].

Our results provide important insight for the development of an anticancer drug for OMM. However, the limitations of this study should be considered. In our in vivo experiments, there was no negative control. When tumor cells were implanted into mice, a tumor mass was usually detected 12–14 days after the initial implantation. If they received no subsequent treatment, the mice died within 2–3 days, largely due to extensive metastasis and weight loss. Our positive control, the cisplatin-only group, also showed a similar trend. Though the xenografted cells mimicked clinical findings, the observations from this study were based on cells from a single case of OMM. OMM is a different disease from skin melanoma. Because OMM is rare, there are very few established OMM cell lines. Further in vitro and in vivo studies using other OMM cells are needed to confirm our current findings. In addition, the association of 4HR and MMP is indirect relation. In case of human umbilical vein endothelial cell and RAW264.7 cell, the administration of 4HR increases the expression level of MMPs via upregulation of TGF-β1. The signaling pathway of TGF-β1 is largely different between normal healthy cell and malignant cell. Thus, the effect of 4HR administration on the expression level of MMP will be different to cellular type.

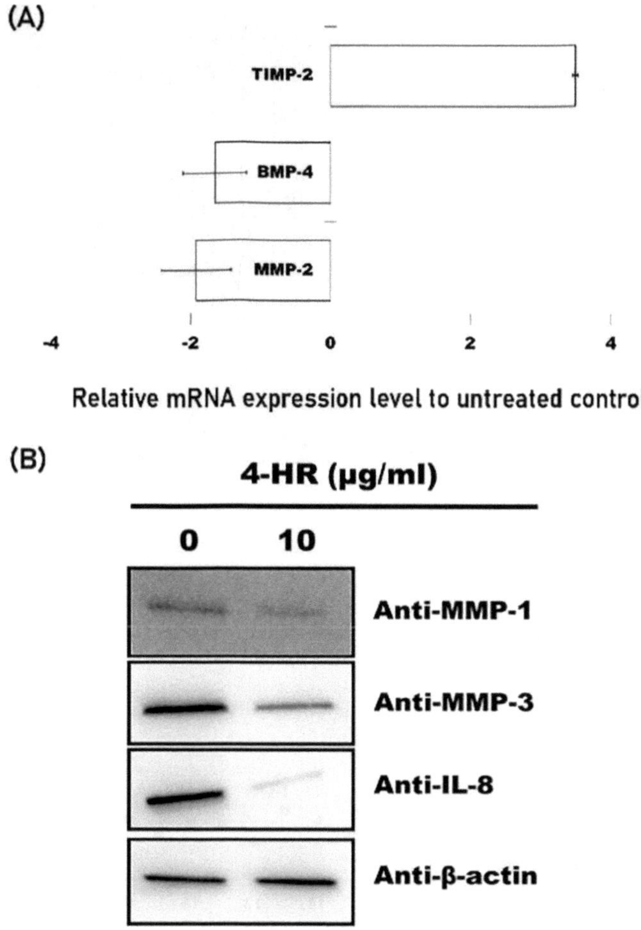

Fig. 3.16 The change of MMP expression by 4HR administration in primary cultured oral malignant melanoma cells. (**a**) Quantitative reverse transcriptase–polymerase chain reaction result. The expression level of MMP-2 mRNA is lower in 4HR group compared to untreated control. (**b**) Western blot result. The expression level of MMP-1 and -3 is much lower in 4HR group compared to untreated control (background data of author's previous publication [82])

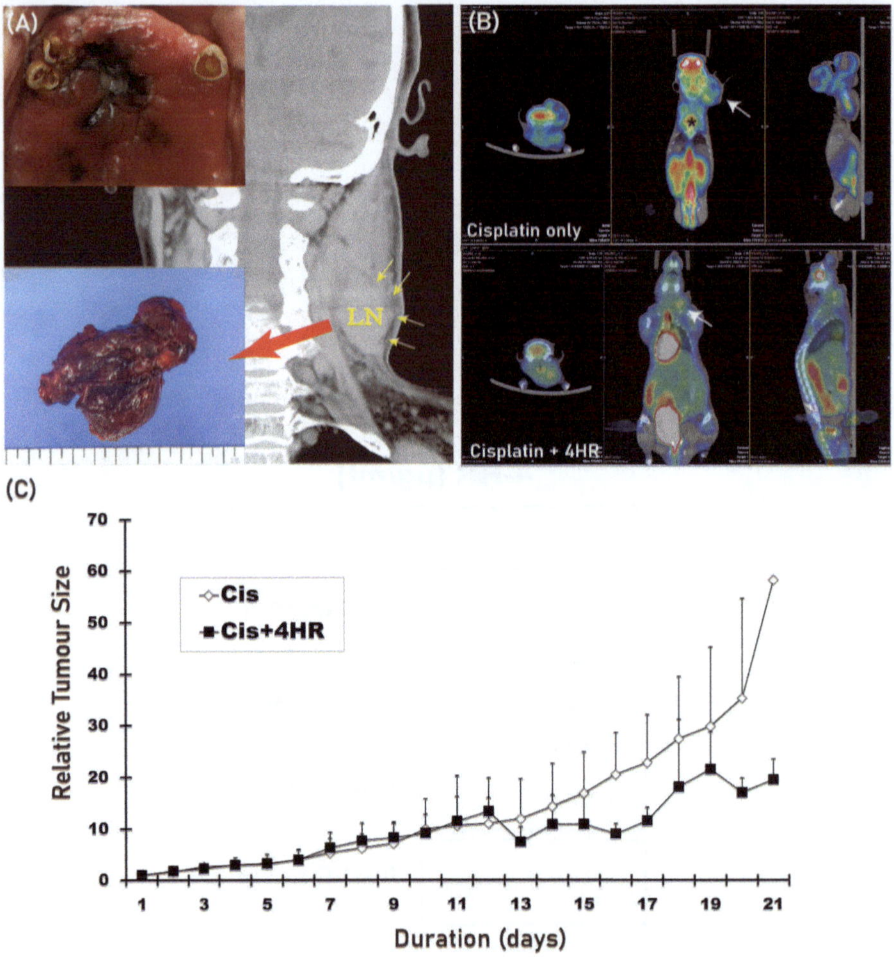

Fig. 3.17 Oral malignant melanoma (OMM). (**a**) Primary lesion of OMM was found in the palate. Patient showed regional lymph node (LN) metastasis (arrows). OMM cells were collected from the excised metastatic LN. (**b**) Primary cultured OMM cells are implanted into the submandibular area. Mass size of cisplatin +4HR group is smaller than that of cisplatin-only group (arrow). Interestingly, body size of cisplatin +4HR group looks much larger than that of cisplatin-only group. LN in the back (asterisk) shows metastasis. (**c**) Relative tumor size is much smaller in cisplatin +4HR group (edited from authors' previous publication [82])

3.6 The Effect of 4HR Administration on Various Tumors

Tumor cells and primary cultured gingival fibroblast are seeded and treated with 4HR, and cell proliferation is assessed by 3-[4,5-dimethylthiazol-2-yl]-2,5 diphenyl tetrazolium bromide (MTT) assay (Fig. 3.18). HepG2 is a cell from hepatoma. H1299 cell is a cell from human non-small-cell lung carcinoma cells. Antiproliferative effects of 4HR are observed at 40 h after 4HR treatment.

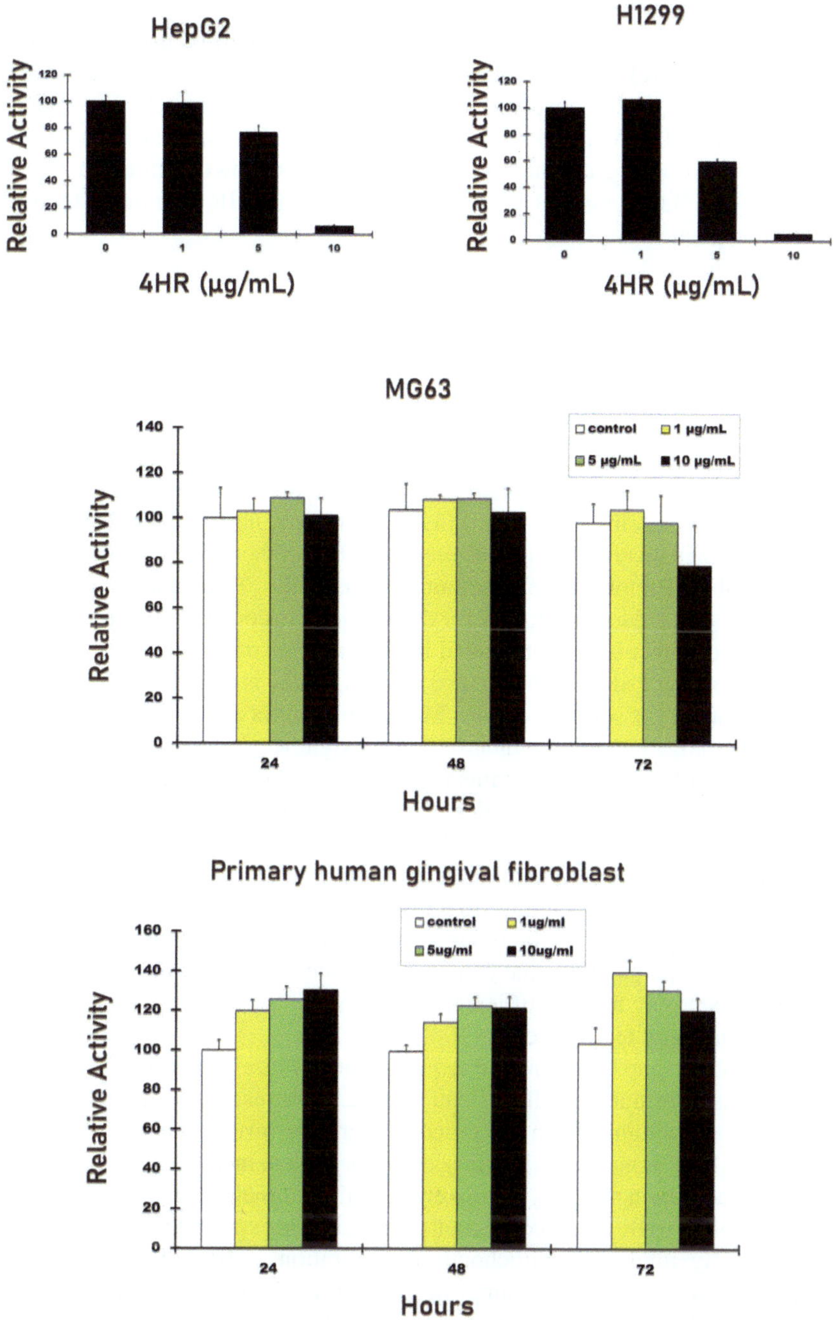

Fig. 3.18 The effect of 4HR administration on various types of cells. The cellular growth suppression is evident for HepG2 and H1299 cell by 4HR administration. However, MG63 and gingival fibroblast receive less impact by 4HR administration (background data of author's previous publication [13])

Additionally, breast cancer cells (MCF-7 and SKBR3) show reduced proliferation by 4HR administration (data not shown). MCF-7 is a cell of estrogen receptor-positive, and SKBR3 is a cell of estrogen receptor-negative breast cancer cell. Reduced viability is also observed in SNU601 gastric cancer cell line after 24-h exposure with 4HR (5 μg/mL). However, MG63 cells (osteosarcoma-like cell) and primary cultured gingival fibroblasts show less growth inhibition by 4HR administration. Based on this preliminary screening, 4HR is more effective on epithelial originated tumors.

3.7 Closing Remark

In this chapter, the anti-tumor effect of 4HR has been reviewed. In the microbiological study [68], the biological effect of 4HR is a species nonspecific. Unlike microorganism, human cells express much many kinds of protein. The three-dimensional conformation of proteins should be different from protein to protein. Evolutionally preserved proteins may have high affinity to 4HR, but the affinity to novel proteins is unpredictable. Tumor has genetic mutation generally. Thus, anti-tumor effect of 4HR should be tested to each tumor for definite conclusion. Tumor species nonspecific anti-tumor effect is not anticipated in 4HR administration.

Administration of 4HR in the context of malignancy is expected to provide benefits to the patient for several reasons. Malignant tumors are characterized by their highly proliferative potential, which requires a significant amount of ATP for fueling the elevated levels of cancer metabolism. Both mitochondrial respiration and glycolysis pathways play crucial roles in providing ATP to support tumor proliferation. Mitochondria, having their own DNA and resembling prokaryotes, are involved in this energy production. The administration of 4HR leads to the suppression of mitochondrial respiration, and this effect is not specific to any cell type. As a result, normal cells compensate for the reduced ATP production by increasing the activation of glycolysis, a pathway that can help generate ATP. However, this compensatory mechanism may not be sufficient for tumor cells with high ATP demands to fulfill their energetic requirements.

This metabolic gap between ATP requirement and its availability can have detrimental effects on tumor cells. It can lead to increased stress on the mitochondria and endoplasmic reticulum, which are crucial organelles involved in maintaining cell homeostasis. Furthermore, the inability of tumor cells to meet their energy demands may trigger cellular apoptosis, ultimately resulting in their death. Accordingly, the administration of 4HR in the context of malignancy is expected to be beneficial for the patient. By inhibiting mitochondrial respiration, 4HR induces a metabolic imbalance in tumor cells that cannot be compensated solely by glycolysis activation. This imbalance leads to increased stress and apoptotic cell death, specifically targeting tumor cells and potentially halting their proliferation.

The binding of 4HR to target protein will change the conformation of the target protein. It may inhibit or activate the target protein. Any drug can change protein conformation can induce the stress of the endoplasmic reticulum. The administration of

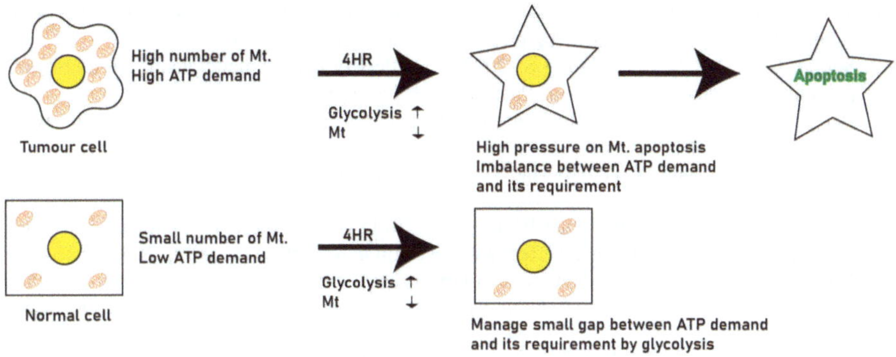

Fig. 3.19 The effect of 4HR administration on cancer metabolism. As 4HR is a chaperone, it can suppress cellular metabolism as cell-type nonspecific manner. 4HR can suppress mitochondrial respiration. Consequently, the administration of 4HR on cancer cell will result in reduced mitochondrial ATP and ROS production. Mitochondrial ROS, which is a by-product of mitochondrial respiration, is a key element for inducing hypoxia-inducible factor (HIF: key element of cancer angiogenesis). Reduced ATP production in the mitochondria can be compensated by accelerated glycolysis in normal cell. However, this compensation is not enough in tumor cell and results in cellular apoptosis

4HR increases endoplasmic reticulum stress [96]. The stress of the endoplasmic reticulum may induce cellular apoptosis. Tumor metabolism is influenced by 4HR administration, too (Fig. 3.19). There are many things that remain unclear. Further study is required to assess the anti-tumor effect of 4HR.

References

1. National Toxicology Program (1988) Toxicology and carcinogenesis studies of 4-hexylresorcinol (CAS no. 136-77-6) in F344/N rats and B6C3F1 mice (gavage studies). Natl Toxicol Program Tech Rep Ser 330:1–166
2. Koshiura RH, Kagotani Y, Ujiie T (1962) Experimental anticancer studies. XVI. Preparation and anticancer activity of 4-amino-6-hexylresorcinol on Ehrlich carcinoma in mice. Chem Pharm Bull 10:528–532
3. Koshimura S, Murasawa K, Nakagawa E, Ueda M, Bando Y, Hirata R (1956) Experimental anticancer studies. II. On the anti-tumor effect of 6-(2′-hydroxy-3′, 5′-dihalophenylazo)-4-hexylresorcinol and related compounds on Yoshida sarcoma and Ehrlich ascites carcinoma in vivo. Gan 47(3–4):393–397
4. Lee IS, Kim DW, Oh JH et al (2021) Effects of 4-hexylresorcinol on craniofacial growth in rats. Int J Mol Sci 22(16):8935
5. He Q, Ma P, Torshizi R (2022) The impact of some natural phenolic compounds on α-glucosidase and sorbitol dehydrogenase enzymes, and anti-leukemia cancer potential, spin density distributions, and in silico studies. J Oleo Sci 71(6):863–873
6. Dieter MP, Jameson CW, French JE et al (1989) Development and validation of a cellular transplant model for leukemia in Fischer rats: a short-term assay for potential anti-leukemic chemicals. Leuk Res 13(9):841–849
7. Haseman JK, Huff JE, Rao GN, Arnold JE, Boorman GA, McConnell EE (1985) Neoplasms observed in untreated and corn oil gavage control groups of F344/N rats and (C57BL/6N X C3H/HeN)F1 (B6C3F1) mice. J Natl Cancer Inst 75(5):975–984

8. Yoon JH, Kim DW, Lee SK, Kim SG (2022) Effects of 4-hexylresorcinol administration on the submandibular glands in a growing rat model. Head Face Med 18:16
9. Sun D, Li X, Nie S, Liu J, Wang S (2023) Disorders of cancer metabolism: the therapeutic potential of cannabinoids. Biomed Pharmacother 157:113993
10. Jiang P, Du W, Wu M (2014) Regulation of the pentose phosphate pathway in cancer. Protein Cell 5(8):592–602
11. Liberti MV, Locasale JW (2016) The Warburg effect: how does it benefit cancer cells? Trends Biochem Sci 41(3):211–218
12. Kim SG, Lee SW, Park YW, Jeong JH, Choi JY (2011) 4-hexylresorcinol inhibits NF-κB phosphorylation and has a synergistic effect with cisplatin in KB cells. Oncol Rep 26(6):1527–1532
13. Kim SG, Choi JY (2013) 4-hexylresorcinol exerts antitumor effects via suppression of calcium oscillation and its antitumor effects are inhibited by calcium channel blockers. Oncol Rep 29(5):1835–1840
14. Kim SG, Kim AS, Jeong JH, Choi JY, Kweon H (2012) 4-hexylresorcinol stimulates the differentiation of SCC-9 cells through the suppression of E2F2, E2F3 and Sp3 expression and the promotion of Sp1 expression. Oncol Rep 28(2):677–681
15. Kang YJ, Yang WG, Chae WS, Kim DW, Kim SG, Rotaru H (2022) Administration of 4-hexylresorcinol increases p53-mediated transcriptional activity in oral cancer cells with the p53 mutation. Oncol Rep 48(3):160
16. Almowallad S, Alqahtani LS, Mobashir M (2022) NF-kB in signaling patterns and its temporal dynamics encode/decode human diseases. Life (Basel) 12(12):2012
17. Gupta SC, Sundaram C, Reuter S, Aggarwal BB (2010) Inhibiting NF-κB activation by small molecules as a therapeutic strategy. Biochim Biophys Acta 1799:775–787
18. Orlowski RZ, Baldwin AS Jr (2002) NF-kappaB as a therapeutic target in cancer. Trends Mol Med 8:385–389
19. Bui JD, Schreiber RD (2007) Cancer immunosurveillance, immunoediting and inflammation: independent or interdependent processes? Curr Opin Immunol 19:203–208
20. Kim SG, Jeong JH, Park YW et al (2011) 4-hexylresorcinol inhibits transglutaminase-2 activity and has synergistic effects along with cisplatin in KB cells. Oncol Rep 25(6):1597–1602
21. Jacobs MD, Harrison SC (1998) Structure of an IkappaBalpha/NF-kappaB complex. Cell 95:749–758
22. Matthews JR, Hay RT (1995) Regulation of the DNA binding activity of NF-κB. Int J Biochem Cell Biol 27:865–879
23. Kim DS, Han BG, Park KS, Lee BI, Kim SY, Bae CD (2010) I-kappaBalpha depletion by transglutaminase 2 and mu-calpain occurs in parallel with the ubiquitin-proteasome pathway. Biochem Biophys Res Commun 399:300–306
24. Mann AP, Verma A, Sethi G et al (2006) Overexpression of tissue transglutaminase leads to constitutive activation of nuclear factor-kappaB in cancer cells: delineation of a novel pathway. Cancer Res 66:8788–8795
25. Piacentini M, Amendola A, Ciccosanti F et al (2005) Type 2 transglutaminase and cell death. Prog Exp Tumor Res 38:58–74
26. Campisi A, Caccamo D, Raciti G et al (2003) Glutamate-induced increases in transglutaminase activity in primary cultures of astroglial cells. Brain Res 978:24–30
27. Ientile R, Caccamo D, Griffin M (2007) Tissue transglutaminase and the stress response. Amino Acids 33:385–394
28. Lee M, Yu S, Lee YS, Park JS (2001) Characterization of nuclear factors binding to AT-rich element in the rat p53 promoter. J Cell Biochem 80:580–588
29. Kubista M, Akerman B, Nordén B (1987) Characterization of interaction between DNA and 4′,6-diamidino-2-phenylindole by optical spectroscopy. Biochemistry 26:4545–4553
30. Barcellona ML, Gratton E (1990) The fluorescence properties of a DNA probe. Eur Biophys J 17:315–323
31. Banerjee D, Pal SK (2008) Dynamics in the DNA recognition by DAPI: exploration of the various binding modes. J Phys Chem B 112:1016–1021

32. Malinge JM, Giraud-Panis MJ, Leng M (1999) Interstrand cross-links of cisplatin induce striking distortions in DNA. J Inorg Biochem 77:23–29
33. Jamshidipour R, Pinho EB, Howell SB (1994) In vivo modulation of cisplatin cytotoxicity by the chelcystokinin antagonist MK-329 in human pancreatic cancer xenografts. Anticancer Res 14:2611–2616
34. Yang LC, Ng DC, Bikle DD (2003) Role of protein kinase Cα in calcium-induced keratinocyte differentiation: defective regulation in squamous cell carcinoma. J Cell Physiol 195:249–259
35. Bezzi P, Carmignoto G, Pasti L et al (1998) Prostaglandins stimulate calcium-dependent glutamate release in astrocytes. Nature 391:281–285
36. Parri HR, Gould TM, Crunelli V (2001) Spontaneous astrocytic Ca2+ oscillations in situ drive NMDAR-mediated neuronal excitation. Nat Neurosci 4:803–812
37. Choi SW, Park SY, Hong SP, Pai H, Choi JY, Kim SG (2004) The expression of NMDA receptor 1 is associated with clinicopathological parameters and prognosis in the oral squamous cell carcinoma. J Oral Pathol Med 33:533–537
38. Rzeski W, Ikonomidou C, Turski L (2002) Glutamate antagonists limit tumor growth. Biochem Pharmacol 64:1195–1200
39. Wong CF, Barnes LM, Dahler AL et al (2005) E2F suppression and Sp1 overexpression are sufficient to induce the differentiation-specific marker, transglutaminase type 1, in a squamous cell carcinoma cell line. Oncogene 24:3525–3534
40. Bruckman KC, Schönleben F, Qiu W, Woo VL, Su GH (2010) Mutational analyses of the BRAF, KRAS, and PIK3CA genes in oral squamous cell carcinoma. Oral Surg Oral Med Oral Pathol Oral Radiol Endod 110:632–637
41. Wong CF, Barnes LM, Dahler AL et al (2003) E2F modulates keratinocyte squamous differentiation: implications for E2F inhibition in squamous cell carcinoma. J Biol Chem 278:28516–28522
42. Wu Z, Zheng S, Yu Q (2009) The E2F family and the role of E2F1 in apoptosis. Int J Biochem Cell Biol 41:2389–2397
43. Polyak K, Kato JY, Solomon MJ et al (1994) p27kip1, a cyclin-Cdk inhibitor, links transforming growth factor-beta and contact inhibition to cell cycle arrest. Genes Dev 8:9–22
44. DeGregori J, Kowalik T, Nevins JR (1995) Cellular targets for activation by the E2F1 transcription factor include DNA synthesis- and G1/S-regulatory genes. Mol Cell Biol 15:4215–4224
45. Wu L, Timmers C, Maiti B et al (2001) The E2F1-3 transcription factors are essential for cellular proliferation. Nature 414:457–462
46. Braig M, Lee S, Loddenkemper C et al (2005) Oncogene-induced senescence as an initial barrier in lymphoma development. Nature 436:660–665
47. Hazar-Rethinam M, Cameron SR, Dahler AL et al (2011) Loss of E2F7 expression is an early event in squamous differentiation and causes derepression of the key differentiation activator Sp1. J Invest Dermatol 131:1077–1084
48. Muller H, Bracken AP, Vernell R et al (2001) E2Fs regulate the expression of genes involved in differentiation, development, proliferation, and apoptosis. Genes Dev 15:267–285
49. Peltonen JK, Helppi HM, Pääkkö P, Turpeenniemi-Hujanen T, Vähäkangas KH (2010) p53 in head and neck cancer: functional consequences and environmental implications of TP53 mutations. Head Neck Oncol 2:36
50. Lindemann A, Takahashi H, Patel A, Osman A, Myers J (2018) Targeting the DNA damage response in OSCC with TP53 mutations. J Dent Res 97(6):635–644
51. Pecorino L (2016) Molecular biology of cancer, 4th edn. Oxford University Press
52. Brooks CL, Gu W (2003) Ubiquitination, phosphorylation and acetylation: the molecular basis for p53 regulation. Curr Opin Cell Biol 15(2):164–171
53. Oren M, Rotter V (2010) Mutant p53 gain-of-function in cancer. Cold Spring Harb Perspect Biol 2(2):a001107
54. Klimovich B, Stiewe T, Timofeev O (2020) Inactivation of Mdm2 restores apoptosis proficiency of cooperativity mutant p53 in vivo. Cell Cycle 19(1):109–123
55. Kanapathipillai M (2018) Treating p53 mutant aggregation-associated cancer. Cancers (Basel) 10(6):154

56. Muller PA, Vousden KH (2014) Mutant p53 in cancer: new functions and therapeutic opportunities. Cancer Cell 25(3):304–317
57. Soussi T, Kato S, Levy PP, Ishioka C (2005) Reassessment of the TP53 mutation database in human disease by data mining with a library of TP53 missense mutations. Hum Mutat 25(1):6–17
58. Lee EJ, Kim J, Lee SA et al (2005) Characterization of newly established oral cancer cell lines derived from six squamous cell carcinoma and two mucoepidermoid carcinoma cells. Exp Mol Med 37(5):379–390
59. de Bakker T, Journe F, Descamps G et al (2022) Restoring p53 function in head and neck squamous cell carcinoma to improve treatments. Front Oncol 11:799993
60. Lambert JM, Gorzov P, Veprintsev DB et al (2009) PRIMA-1 reactivates mutant p53 by covalent binding to the core domain. Cancer Cell 15(5):376–388
61. Chen HM, Lee YH, Wang YJ (2015) ROS-triggered signaling pathways involved in the cytotoxicity and tumor promotion effects of pentachlorophenol and tetrachlorohydroquinone. Chem Res Toxicol 28(3):339–350
62. Yao T-P, Seto E (2011) Histone deacetylases: the biology and clinical implication, vol 206. Springer Science & Business Media
63. Paluvai H, Di Giorgio E, Brancolini C (2018) Unscheduled HDAC4 repressive activity in human fibroblasts triggers TP53-dependent senescence and favors cell transformation. Mol Oncol 12(12):2165–2181
64. Kim SG (2022) 4-hexylresorcinol: pharmacologic chaperone and its application for wound healing. Maxillofac Plast Reconstr Surg 44:5
65. Lee IS, Chang JH, Kim DW, Kim SG, Kim TW (2021) The effect of 4-hexylresorinol administration on NAD+ level and SIRT activity in Saos-2 cells. Maxillofac Plast Reconstr Surg 43:39
66. Kim JY, Kweon HY, Kim DW, Choi JY, Kim SG (2021) 4-hexylresorcinol inhibits class I histone deacetylases in human umbilical cord endothelial cells. Appl Sci 11(8):3486
67. Kim DW, Jo YY, Garagiola U, Choi JY, Kang YJ, Oh JH, Kim SG (2020) Increased level of vascular endothelial growth factors by 4-hexylresorcinol is mediated by transforming growth factor-β1 and accelerates capillary regeneration in the burns in diabetic animals. Int J Mol Sci 21(10):3473
68. El-Registan GI, Mulyukin AL, Nikolaev YA, Stepanenko IY, Kozlova AN, Martirosova EI, Shanenko EF, Strakhovskaya MG, Revina AA (2005) The role of microbial low-molecular-weight autoregulatory factors (alkylhydroxybenzenes) in resistance of microorganisms to radiation and heat shock. Adv Space Res 36(9):1718–1728
69. Kang YJ, Kim DW, Che X, Choi JY, Kim SG (2022) Inhibition of TP53 mutant oral cancer by reactivating p53. Appl Sci 12(12):5921
70. Buonocore G, Perrone S, Tataranno ML (2010) Oxygen toxicity: chemistry and biology of reactive oxygen species, vol 15. Elsevier, pp 186–190
71. Yen GC, Duh PD, Lin CW (2003) Effects of resveratrol and 4-hexylresorcinol on hydrogen peroxide-induced oxidative DNA damage in human lymphocytes. Free Radic Res 37(5):509–514
72. Guandalini E, Ioppolo A, Mantovani A, Stacchini P, Giovannini C (1998) 4-hexylresorcinol as inhibitor of shrimp melanosis: efficacy and residues studies; evaluation of possible toxic effect in a human intestinal in vitro model (Caco-2); preliminary safety assessment. Food Addit Contam 15(2):171–180
73. Thiagarajan D, Vedantham S, Ananthakrishnan R, Schmidt AM, Ramasamy R (2016) Mechanisms of transcription factor acetylation and consequences in hearts. Biochim Biophys Acta 1862(12):2221–2231
74. Jimenez GS, Khan SH, Stommel JM, Wahl GM (1999) p53 regulation by post-translational modification and nuclear retention in response to diverse stresses. Oncogene 18(53):7656–7665
75. Stock AM, Robinson VL, Goudreau PN (2000) Two-component signal transduction. Annu Rev Biochem 69:183–215

76. Chia J, Tham KM, Gill DJ, Bard-Chapeau EA, Bard FA (2014) ERK8 is a negative regulator of O-GalNAc glycosylation and cell migration. elife 3:e01828
77. Tanaka N, Mimura M, Ogi K et al (2004) Primary malignant melanoma of the oral cavity: assessment of outcome from the clinical records of 35 patients. Int J Oral Maxillofac Surg 33:761–765
78. Mücke T, Hölzle F, Kesting MR et al (2009) Tumor size and depth in primary malignant melanoma in the oral cavity influences survival. J Oral Maxillofac Surg 67:1409–1415
79. Vikey AK, Vikey D (2012) Primary malignant melanoma of head and neck: a comprehensive review of literature. Oral Oncol 48:399–403
80. Rapini RP, Golitz LE, Greer RO et al (1985) Primary malignant melanoma of the oral cavity. A review of 177 cases. Cancer 55:1543–1551
81. Nayak MT, Singh A, Mathur RM et al (2012) Second primary oral melanoma: a rare presentation. J Oral Maxillofac Pathol 16:88–90
82. Lee SW, Kim SG, Park YW, Kweon H, Kim JY, Rotaru H (2013) Cisplatin and 4-hexylresorcinol synergise to decrease metastasis and increase survival rate in an oral mucosal melanoma xenograft model: a preliminary study. Tumour Biol 34(3):1595–1603
83. Lens MB, Eisen TG (2003) Systemic chemotherapy in the treatment of malignant melanoma. Expert Opin Pharmacother 4:2205–2211
84. Beguerie JR, Xingzhong J, Valdez RP (2010) Tamoxifen vs. non-tamoxifen treatment for advanced melanoma: a meta-analysis. Int J Dermatol 49:1194–1202
85. Hodi FS, Friedlander P, Corless CL et al (2008) Major response to imatinib mesylate in KIT-mutated melanoma. J Clin Oncol 26:2046–2051
86. Tanaka T, Nakayama H, Yoshitake Y et al (2012) Selective inhibition of nuclear factor-κB by nuclear factor-κB essential modulator-binding domain peptide suppresses the metastasis of highly metastatic oral squamous cell carcinoma. Cancer Sci 103:455–463
87. Kim SG, Song JY (2012) Therapeutic targeting of oncogenic transforming growth factor-β1 signaling by antisense oligonucleotides in oral squamous cell carcinoma. Oncol Rep 28:539–544
88. Yang X, Ren GX, Zhang CP et al (2010) Neck dissection and post-operative chemotherapy with dimethyl triazeno imidazole carboxamide and cisplatin protocol are useful for oral mucosal melanoma. BMC Cancer 10:623
89. Umeda M, Komatsubara H, Shigeta T et al (2008) Treatment and prognosis of malignant melanoma of the oral cavity: preoperative surgical procedure increases risk of distant metastasis. Oral Surg Oral Med Oral Pathol Oral Radiol Endod 106:51–57
90. Lin YS, Chuang MT, Chen CH et al (2012) Nicotinic acid hydroxamate downregulated the melanin synthesis and tyrosinase activity through activating the MEK/ERK and AKT/GSK3β signaling pathways. J Agric Food Chem 60:4859–4864
91. Chen QX, Ke LN, Song KK et al (2004) Inhibitory effects of hexylresorcinol and dodecylresorcinol on mushroom (Agaricus bisporus) tyrosinase. Protein J 23:135–141
92. McLean N, Tighiouart M, Muller S (2008) Primary mucosal melanoma of the head and neck. Comparison of clinical presentation and histopathologic features of oral and sinonasal melanoma. Oral Oncol 44:1039–1046
93. Meleti M, Leemans CR, de Bree R et al (2008) Head and neck mucosal melanoma: experience with 42 patients, with emphasis on the role of postoperative radiotherapy. Head Neck 30:1543–1551
94. Wennerberg J, Biörklund A, Tropé C (1988) The effect of cisplatin and fluorouracil on xenografted human squamous cell carcinoma of the head and neck. Arch Otolaryngol Head Neck Surg 114:162–167
95. Johnsson A, Olsson C, Nygren O et al (1995) Pharmacokinetics and tissue distribution of cisplatin in nude mice: platinum levels and cisplatin-DNA adducts. Cancer Chemother Pharmacol 37:23–31
96. Kim JY, Kim DW, Lee SK, Choi JY, Che X, Kim SG, Garagiola U (2021) Increased expression of TGF-β1 by 4-hexylresorcinol is mediated by endoplasmic reticulum and mitochondrial stress in human umbilical endothelial vein cells. Appl Sci 11:9128

Chapter 4
Antioxidant and Anti-Inflammatory Activity of 4-Hexylresorcinol

Abstract This chapter discusses the role of 4HR ointment in dental injury treatment and its potential to reduce oxidative stress and inflammation. Dental procedures can induce oxidative stress, leading to an increase in pro-inflammatory molecules such as TNF-α and IL1β. Antioxidants like 4HR can alleviate oxidative stress and facilitate tissue healing. The study found that 4HR treatment reduced hydrogen peroxide-induced oxidative stress in dental pulp cells, decreased expression levels of TNF-α and IL1β, and improved total antioxidant capacity and GPx levels. In a tooth fracture model, 4HR application resulted in fewer blood clots and better cellular regeneration, indicating its potential to support dental pulp tissue repair. The chapter concludes that 4HR ointment shows promise in reducing oxidative stress and downregulating inflammatory cytokine expression, which may improve therapeutic outcomes. Further investigation using other models is warranted.

Keywords 4-hexylresorcinol (4HR) · Dental injury · Oxidative stress · Inflammation · Antioxidant

Reactive oxygen species (ROS) are chemical compounds that are highly reactive and can damage cells and tissues in the human body [1]. These compounds are primarily produced by the mitochondria, which are the powerhouses of the cells [2]. The mitochondria are responsible for producing ATP, the main source of energy for cells, through a process called oxidative respiration that uses glucose. During this process, ROS is generated as a by-product of the reaction [3]. ROS can be likened to the waste produced by a factory during production, and if not properly disposed of, it can cause damage to the environment. Similarly, if ROS is not neutralized by antioxidants, it can damage cells, proteins, and DNA, leading to oxidative stress and a range of diseases.

Cells have evolved their own protective mechanisms to prevent oxidative damage by scavenging ROS and maintaining cellular homeostasis [4]. These mechanisms involve a range of endogenous antioxidant systems, including enzymes like

S.-G. Kim, *Biomedical Application of 4-Hexylresorcinol*,
https://doi.org/10.1007/978-981-97-0637-2_4

superoxide dismutase (SOD), glutathione reductase, glutathione peroxidase (GPx), glutathione S-transferase, and catalase (CAT) [5].

SOD catalyzes the conversion of the highly reactive superoxide radical to the less harmful hydrogen peroxide (H_2O_2), which is then further detoxified by GPx and CAT [6, 7]. GPx utilizes glutathione as a cofactor to reduce H_2O_2 and organic hydroperoxides to water and alcohol, respectively [8]. CAT catalyzes the breakdown of H_2O_2 into water and oxygen (Fig. 4.1). Glutathione S-transferase also plays an important role in detoxifying xenobiotics and other harmful substances [9, 10].

Together, these antioxidant enzymes form the first line of defense against oxidative stress [4, 5]. By neutralizing ROS and converting them into less reactive and harmless forms, these systems prevent cellular damage, dysfunction, and inflammation. Therefore, the proper functioning of these endogenous antioxidant systems is crucial for maintaining cellular homeostasis and preventing oxidative damage.

The natural resources contain various antioxidant compounds that can be used to reduce oxidative stress [11, 12]. These compounds can be consumed as food ingredients [13] or health supplements [14]. Among the various phenolic compounds, 4-hexylresorcinol (4HR) stands out as it has both antioxidant and anti-inflammatory properties [15, 16]. 4HR is a resorcinolic lipid and phenolic compound that is known to possess strong antioxidant properties [17]. Therefore, it can be used to effectively reduce oxidative stress and inflammation.

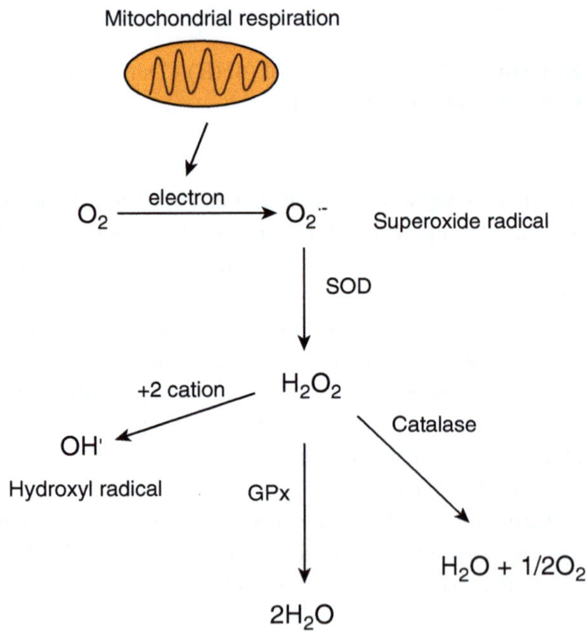

Fig. 4.1 The production of ROS is started from electron leakage of mitochondria or enzyme reaction. Superoxide radical is converted to hydrogen peroxide by superoxide dismutase (SOD). Subsequently, hydrogen peroxide can be processed by glutathione peroxidase (GPx) or catalase. If hydrogen peroxide has undergone through Fenton reaction, highly reactive hydroxyl radical is produced. It can cause cellular damage

4.1 Antioxidant Property of 4HR

Endogenous ROS is mainly produced by the mitochondria and plays a crucial role in normal cellular physiology. However, ROS production can be excessive under certain conditions such as high levels of glucose, exposure to toxins, and carcinogenesis. High glucose levels are closely associated with diabetes, and the effects of 4-h administration of ROS on a diabetic model will be discussed in Chap. 8. In the case of tumor cells, the activation of glycolysis and lactate dehydrogenase, along with the restriction of mitochondrial respiration, may be a survival strategy to alleviate ROS-induced stress and enable faster ATP production.

The increased level of ROS is widely associated with inflammation, and various agents can induce ROS when applied [18]. Bacterial toxin, such as lipopolysaccharide (LPS), hydrogen peroxide, and insect proteins, such as silk sericin, are examples of agents that can induce ROS. Studies have found that the relative SOD levels in response to LPS treatment are significantly lower than those in response to corresponding concentrations of silk sericin, indicating that silk sericin is a much weaker inflammation inducer compared to LPS [19]. The application of ROS-inducing agents can also invite M1-type macrophages, which are known to generate high levels of ROS [18]. In contrast, M2-like macrophages, which are associated with tissue remodeling, have lower levels of ROS than M1-like macrophages [20] (Fig. 4.2).

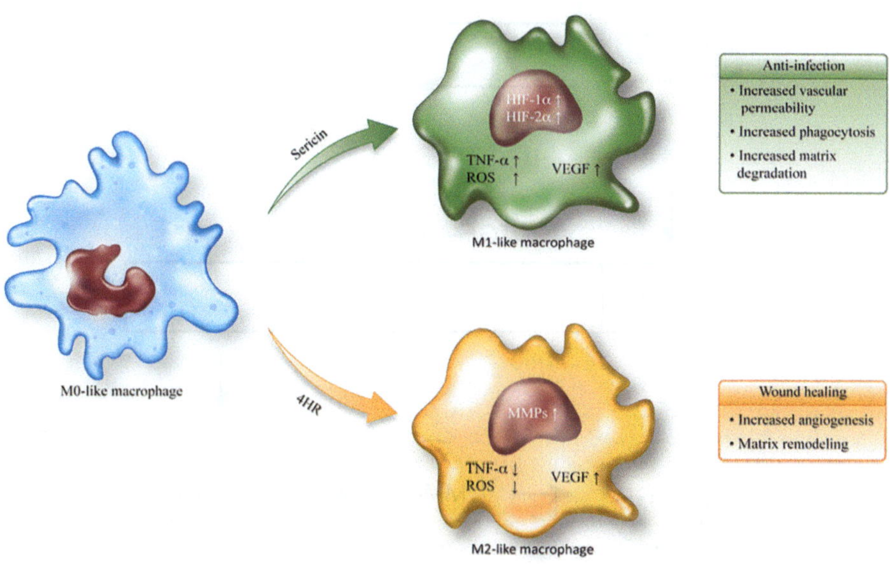

Fig. 4.2 Macrophage polarization by 4HR administration (reproduced from author's previous publication [19])

Several studies have demonstrated the antioxidant properties of 4HR. 4HR inhibits flavonol oxidation [21]. Furthermore, 4HR administration in human lymphocytes reduces hydrogen peroxide-induced DNA damage [22]. Additionally, the administration of 4HR decreases ROS levels induced by hydrogen peroxide pretreatment in RAW264.7 cells [19]. Furthermore, the relative total antioxidant capacity after hydrogen peroxide treatment was significantly higher in 4HR treatment group compared to the untreated control group [19]. 4HR significantly increases GPx activity at 5 μg/mL and 10 μg/mL compared to the untreated control group in RAW264.7 cells receiving hydrogen peroxide pretreatment [19] (Fig. 4.3).

Macrophages are important players in inflammation and remodeling processes. M1-type macrophages are known to be involved in inflammation, while M2-type macrophages are involved in remodeling [18, 23]. Treatment of RAW264.7 cells

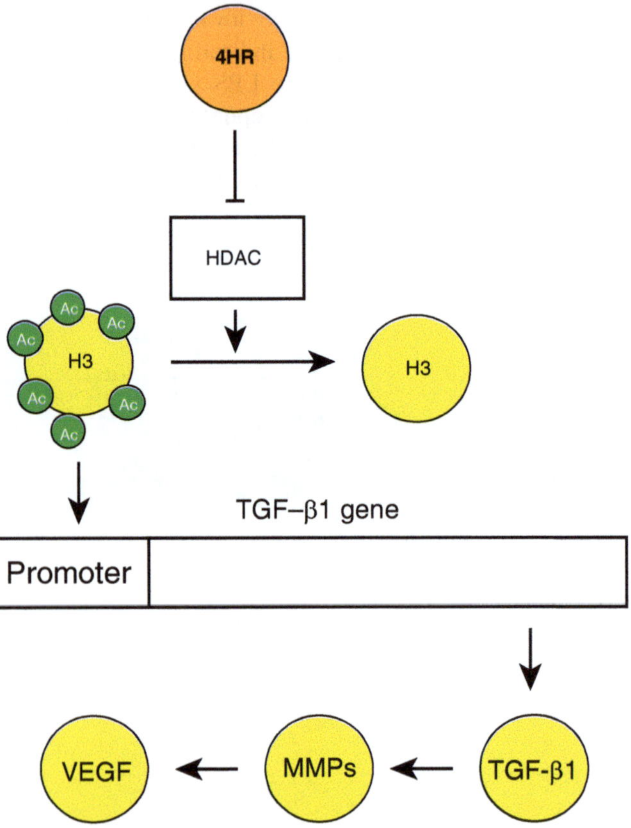

Fig. 4.3 4HR-induced VEGF expression. *ac* acetylation, *H3* histone 3. 4HR is histone deacetylase (HDAC) inhibitor. Hyper-acetylated H3 can bind to TGF-β1 gene promoter and accelerate its transcription and elevate the expression level of TGF-β1. 4HR-induced TGF-β1 can increase the expression level of vascular endothelial growth factor (VEGF) via TGF-β1/matrix metalloproteinase (MMP) axis. This type of angiogenesis is HIF-independent pathway

with 10 μg/mL silk sericin has been found to increase expression of M1 markers such as CD68 and pStat1 [19]. Additionally, treatment of RAW264.7 cells with 10 μg/mL 4HR increased expression of M2 markers such as CD206 and cellular muscular aponeurotic fibrosarcoma (c-Maf) [19]. Sericin has also been found to increase expression of tumor necrosis factor-α (TNF-α) in a dose-dependent manner [24]. Furthermore, exposure to TNF-α has been shown to increase hypoxia-inducible factor-1α (HIF-1α) expression in macrophages under normoxic conditions [25]. Additionally, both sericin and LPS have been observed to increase the levels of ROS in RAW264.7 cells [19]. However, administration of sericin has been found to decrease SOD activity [19] and increase the expression of HIF [19]. It has been suggested that activation of HIF by sericin administration may be mediated by increased ROS production, as ROS are required for TNF-α-mediated stabilization of HIF-1α [26]. Additionally, some molecules, such as LPS, have been found to increase the half-life of HIF via direct stabilization, and these molecules are typically pro-inflammatory [27].

The expression of vascular endothelial growth factor (VEGF) can be modulated by various factors, such as HIF inhibitors and antioxidants. Phenethyl isothiocyanate, a HIF inhibitor, was found to inhibit sericin-induced but not 4HR-induced VEGF expression [19]. On the other hand, 4HR acts as an antioxidant by activating antioxidant enzymes and does not increase the expression of HIF [19]. However, it can increase the expression of matrix metalloproteinases (MMPs), which can regulate the expression level of VEGF by inducing the release of VEGF from the matrix in tumors [28]. Specifically, 4HR-induced VEGF expression requires multiple MMPs, including MMP-2, MMP-3, MMP-9, MMP-13, and MMP-14 [19].

PD166793, an MMP inhibitor, was found to inhibit the expression of MMPs and VEGF induced by 4HR, suggesting the involvement of MMPs in this process [19]. The administration of 4HR increases the expression level of MMP-13 and MMP-14 [19]. However, the MMP-2-only inhibitor could not decrease the 4HR-induced VEGF expression [19]. PD166793 at a dose of 20 nM inhibited the expression of MMP-13 and VEGF induced by 4HR [19]. PD166793 inhibited the expression of MMP-2 and MMP-3 at a lower concentration than that required to inhibit MMP-13 [29]. Therefore, a dose of 20 nM of PD1666793 was sufficient to inhibit these MMPs.

Additionally, TGF-β1, a cytokine, was found to be a key factor for 4HR-induced VEGF expression, and its inhibition can decrease the expression level of 4HR-induced VEGF [30]. As 4HR is a histone deacetylase inhibitor, it can increase the expression level of TGF-β1 via hyperacetylation of histone 3 [30]. TGF-β1 can also increase the expression level of multiple MMPs [31, 32].

In conclusion, 4HR-induced VEGF expression is modulated by multiple factors, including HIF inhibitors, antioxidants, MMPs, and TGF-β1, which can interact in complex ways to regulate VEGF expression. These findings provide insights into the underlying mechanisms of VEGF regulation and suggest potential therapeutic targets for modulating VEGF expression in various disease contexts.

4.2 The Application of 4HR Ointment on Burns

The process of wound healing in burn injuries is a complex and intricate process that involves interactions between cells and the extracellular matrix [33, 34]. However, the treatment of burn patients is complicated by factors such as inflammatory cytokines. Epidermal burn injuries are associated with the expression of many inflammatory cytokines, including tumor necrosis factor-α (TNF-α) [35]. The dysregulation of TNF-α expression has also been linked to sudden infant death syndrome [36]. Experimental burn trauma has been shown to result in a significant increase in TNF-α expression [37]. Attenuation of TNF-α expression by simvastatin application has been found to reduce burn-induced cellular apoptosis and mortality [38].

In summary, the wound healing process in burn injuries is complex and involves various factors, including inflammatory cytokines like TNF-α. The dysregulation of TNF-α expression can have severe consequences, but its attenuation through simvastatin application can reduce the cellular damage and mortality associated with burn injuries. These findings highlight potential targets for therapeutic interventions to improve burn patient outcomes.

The role of TNF-α in regulating burn wound healing has been widely reported in the literature. In one study, it was found that the protein level of TNF-α in cultured RAW264.7 cells was inhibited by 4HR at concentrations ranging from 1 to 10 μg/mL, as evidenced by Western blot analysis (Fig. 4.4) [39].

Lanolin oil serves as the base material for 4HR ointment, which can be prepared in concentrations of 0.2 wt% or 2 wt% for the treatment of burns. The application of 4HR ointment has been shown to accelerate skin wound healing, with a significantly smaller residual defect area observed in the 4HR ointment group compared to the control group at 14 days after burn injury ($P < 0.05$). In addition, the ointment containing 4HR promotes rapid epithelization and reduces the expression of TNF-α (Fig. 4.5). Histological analysis has revealed more evident collagen regeneration in the 4HR groups (Fig. 4.5).

TNF-α is highly expressed in burn wounds, and its prolonged expression is associated with delayed wound healing and local tissue destruction [40]. Statins, such as

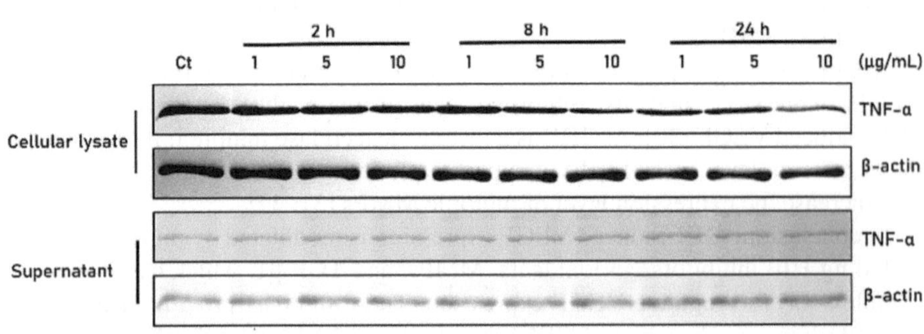

Fig. 4.4 The expression level of TNF-α in RAW264.7 cells after 4HR administration (edited from author's previous publication [39])

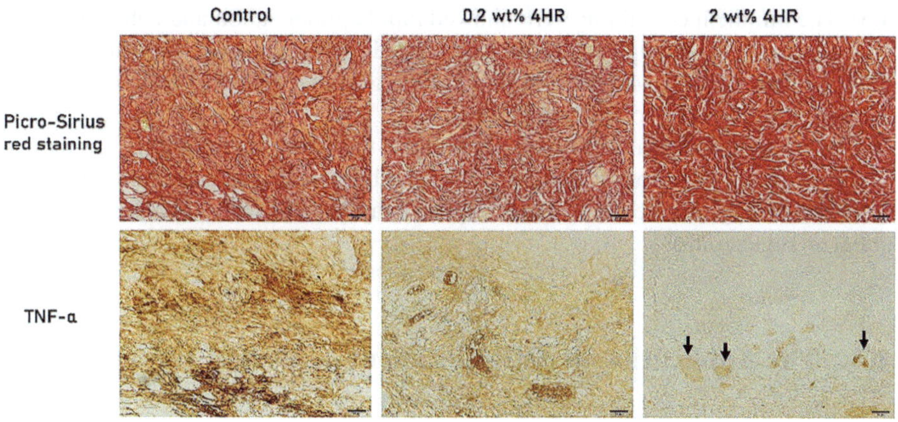

Fig. 4.5 Histological images of burns in the animal model. The red color by Picro-Sirius red staining indicates collagen. The intensity of red color is much enhanced in 2 wt% 4HR group. The expression level of TNF-α is low in 2 wt% 4HR group. TNF-α-positive areas in 2 wt% 4HR group are localized in the vascular channel (arrows) (edited from author's previous publication [39])

simvastatin, have been effective in treating coronary heart disease [41] and are being considered for use as anticancer drugs [42]. Simvastatin has been shown to inhibit TNF-α expression and is considered as a potential treatment for burn wounds [38]. However, the antimicrobial properties of simvastatin have not been reported. Antimicrobial properties are important in burn wound dressings, as the epithelial barrier is destroyed in burn patients [43]. Therefore, if simvastatin is to be used in burn wound dressings due to its TNF-α inhibiting effect, it should be used in combination with an antimicrobial agent.

Silver has been a popular antimicrobial agent used in burn wound care ointments due to its broad spectrum of antibacterial activity and efficacy against resistant microbial strains [44–46]. Silver is easily mixed with ointment bases and has been shown to have favorable clinical results [47]. However, silver-containing dressings, including those based on silver nanoparticles, can lead to silver deposits in burn scar tissue and result in blue or slate-gray skin staining [48]. Although this staining is reported as a transient phenomenon, brown-black pigmentation induced by silver nanoparticles never disappears [48]. Moreover, silver nanoparticles have been linked to immunotoxicity in adult zebrafish [49] and neuronal degeneration in rats [50]. Additionally, silver nanoparticles may induce apoptosis in some cell types via toll-like receptor-mediated pathways [51]. The safety of silver nanoparticles is still controversial for burn wound care, given that their small particle size may enable them to travel to any part of the body, and their metabolic pathways are unclear [52].

4HR has the potential to be an excellent alternative to other ingredients in burn wound care due to its broad antibacterial spectrum and well-known antiseptic properties [53, 54]. Its hydrophobic nature also allows for easy incorporation into lipid-based materials for use in burn wound care ointments [55]. Moreover, this study revealed a previously unknown property of 4HR - TNF-α inhibition (Figs. 4.4 and

4.5). The ointment containing 4HR showed rapid epithelization and collagen regeneration with TNF-α suppression when compared to the control group that used only the base material (Fig. 4.5). These findings suggest that 4HR has great potential as a component in burn wound care ointments.

In summary, the results of this study indicate that 4HR has the ability to suppress TNF-α expression in both RAW264.7 cells and burn wounds. As a result, the use of 4HR-containing ointments on burn wounds may lead to faster epithelization and collagen regeneration.

4.3 The Application of 4HR Ointment on Dental Injury

The dental pulp tissue serves as an initial indicator of dental stress. Various dental treatments can cause stress on the teeth, including the removal of hard tissue in operative dentistry or orthodontic tooth movement during orthodontic treatment [56]. Orthodontic treatment, like other dental procedures, can induce oxidative stress that upregulates the expression of pro-inflammatory molecules such as TNF-α and interleukin-1β (IL1β) [57]. The extent and intensity of oxidative stress determine whether it results in tissue regeneration or necrosis [58]. Therefore, administration of antioxidants is crucial to alleviate excessive oxidative stress and facilitate the healing process.

ROS can be generated as a result of inflammation, and cells synthesize antioxidants to neutralize their harmful effects [59]. Inadequate control of oxidative stress may result in several pathophysiological disorders [60]. ROS stress may damage various organic components, such as proteins and DNA, in the dental pulp tissue [61]. In diabetic individuals, high blood sugar levels increase ROS production and facilitate the development of dental disorders [62]. The endoplasmic reticulum and mitochondria generate many enzymes, including GPx, which minimize ROS production [63].

There are several models available to simulate oxidative stress, including the classic in vitro model using hydrogen peroxide for cellular experiments [65]. In vivo models of dental pulp stress can also be used, such as the application of heavy orthodontic force or the removal of hard dental tissues. These models often induce the expression of pro-inflammatory factors like TNF-α and IL-1β in response to oxidative stress [66].

To promote proper repair of dental pulp tissue, it is important to transiently activate the inflammatory response, which suggests that ROS inducers should also be transient [64]. Antioxidants may help to ensure better tissue regeneration in the face of ROS stress [67]. In fact, treatment with 4HR alleviated hydrogen peroxide-induced oxidative stress in dental pulp cells, resulting in decreased expression levels of TNF-α and IL1β (Fig. 4.6). Furthermore, topical application of 4HR ointment on exposed dental pulp also reduced the expression levels of TNF-α and IL1β [64]. Treatment with 4HR also significantly reduced the levels of total antioxidant capacity (TAC) and GPx compared to ointment base-only values ($P < 0.05$) [64] (Fig. 4.7).

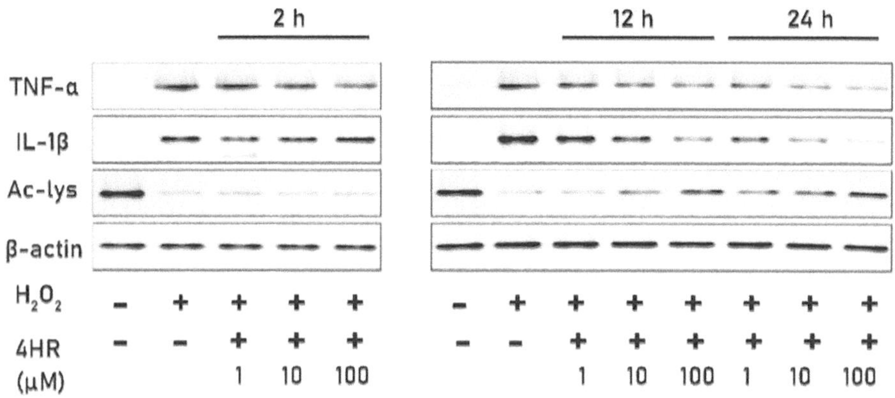

Fig. 4.6 Western blot image in primary cultured rat dental pulp cells from the incisor. Application of hydrogen peroxide increases expression level of TNF-α and IL-1β. The administration of 4HR attenuates hydrogen peroxide-induced inflammatory cytokines (TNF-α and IL-1β). Interestingly, the hydrogen peroxide pretreatment decreases the expression level of acetylated protein (Ac-lys). The suppression of protein acetylation is recovered by 4HR administration (unpublished data from our previous study [64])

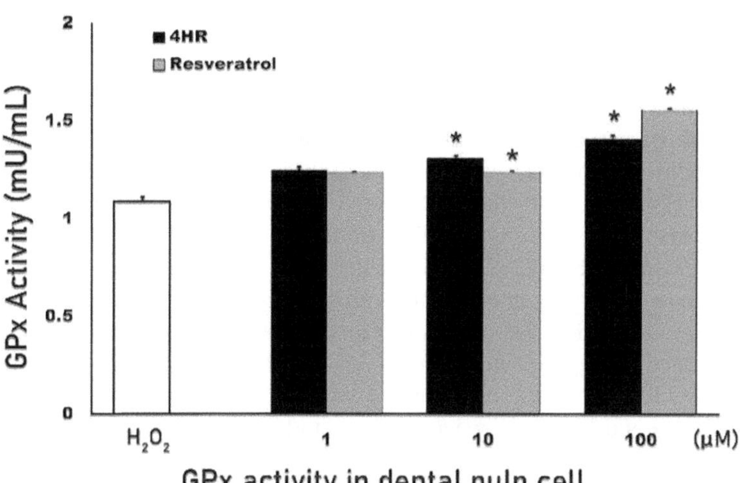

Fig. 4.7 The glutathione peroxidase (GPx) activity in the primary cultured dental pulp cell. The primary dental pulp cells are treated by hydrogen peroxide first. Then, they receive either 4HR or resveratrol. The GPx activity is increased by either 4HR treatment or resveratrol treatment (*$P < 0.05$ compared to hydrogen peroxide treatment only) (modified graph from our previous study [64])

Stress applied to teeth can take different forms, such as dental caries, periodontitis, tooth fracture, orthodontic tooth movement, or cavity preparation [67, 68]. In response, dental pulp produces ROS and triggers an inflammatory reaction [68]. ROS in the inflammatory area alters blood flow in the pulp, contributing to tissue damage [69]. Tooth fracture is a common dental injury that may expose the pulp and cause increased inflammation and edema [70, 71]. Antioxidants can help reverse the inflammatory process and support tissue healing. In this study, we used an incisor cutting model to simulate crown fracture. The group treated with ointment base-only showed massive hemorrhage and blood clots in the pulp, with poor cellular regeneration [64]. However, the application of 4HR reduced the number of blood clots and improved cellular regeneration, indicating its potential to support dental pulp tissue repair.

The increased production of ROS induced by hydrogen peroxide in cell culture models was utilized to assess the potential of our antioxidant screening test. The enzymes CAT, GPx, and SOD play an important role in protecting cells from oxidative damage [72]. Cardiomyocytes treated with hydrogen peroxide have shown a reduction in SOD, CAT, and GPx activity when compared to the untreated control [65]. In our study, pretreatment with 4HR or resveratrol provided protection against oxidative damage in pulp cells [64]. GPx activity and TAC were significantly upregulated when compared to the no pretreatment group ($P < 0.05$) [64]. Resveratrol and 4HR at 10–100 μM increased glutathione levels and GPx activity in human lymphocytes after hydrogen peroxide stimulation [22], similar effects were observed in human umbilical endothelial cells [19]. Reducing oxidative stress can reduce the production of inflammatory cytokines, thus decreasing the availability of various signaling factors, including TNF-α and IL-1β [73].

There are differences in the activity of antioxidant enzymes between animal and cellular models [64]. In the 4HR group, the levels of TAC and GPx are significantly lower than those in the ointment base-only group ($P < 0.05$) [64]. In chronic inflammatory conditions, antioxidant enzyme activity is often elevated due to persistent ROS levels [74, 75]. Both the 4HR-treated and ointment base-only groups show elevated levels of GPx activity and TAC (relative activity >1) compared to the non-injured pulp control [64]. CAT activity is increased in inflamed dental pulp [74], but the application of antioxidants can neutralize ROS and decrease GPx and TAC in the pulp [75]. Antioxidant application may promote early resolution of inflammation in inflamed tissues. The injured dental pulp exhibits chronic inflammation [64], and increased ROS production stimulates the production of inflammatory cytokines such as TNF-α and IL-1β. However, in this study, the expression levels of TNF-α and IL-1β decrease after application of the 4HR ointment [64], which is consistent with in vitro data.

The application of 4HR ointment on the exposed dental pulp results in a reduction of ROS and inflammatory cytokines such as TNF-α and IL1β [64]. Similar studies have shown that 4HR ointment application reduces TNF-α expression and promotes epithelialization in deep burn models and increases capillary regeneration in diabetic animal models [30, 39]. Ointment application is a simple and practical method for dental interventions. However, this study has some limitations. Rat mandibular incisors are relatively large and constantly exposed to the external environment, making long-term observations difficult due to their rapid eruption velocity [76]. This feature of the rat model differs significantly from the human system. Despite this limitation, the application of 4HR has demonstrated benefits in reducing oxidative stress and downregulating inflammatory cytokine expression, which may improve therapeutic outcomes. Therefore, further investigation using other models is warranted based on these promising results.

4.4 Closing Remark

Studies have shown that 4HR exhibits antioxidant activity similar to that of resveratrol. Moreover, 4HR has demonstrated anti-inflammatory effects in burn and dental injuries, indicating its potential in wound healing, prevention of diabetic complications, and tissue engineering. However, to fully comprehend the mechanisms of 4HR's antioxidant and anti-inflammatory effects, further research is necessary to identify possible safety concerns and limitations. Determining the optimal dose and duration of 4HR administration for specific conditions is critical. Moreover, the safety of long-term 4HR use in humans requires further investigation. Despite these limitations, early research shows promising results, indicating that 4HR may serve as a therapeutic agent in various contexts. Future research may explore the synergistic effects of 4HR in combination with other antioxidants or anti-inflammatory agents to enhance its potential benefits.

References

1. Santhakumar AB, Bulmer AC, Singh I (2014) A review of the mechanisms and effectiveness of dietary polyphenols in reducing oxidative stress and thrombotic risk. J Hum Nutr Diet 27(1):1–21
2. Kuo CL, Ponneri Babuharisankar A, Lin YC et al (2022) Mitochondrial oxidative stress in the tumor microenvironment and cancer immunoescape: foe or friend? J Biomed Sci 29:74
3. Zhao RZ, Wang XB, Jiang S et al (2020) Elevated ROS depress mitochondrial oxygen utilization efficiency in cardiomyocytes during acute hypoxia. Pflugers Arch 472(11):1619–1630
4. Ung L, Pattamatta U, Carnt N, Wilkinson-Berka JL, Liew G, White AJR (2017) Oxidative stress and reactive oxygen species: a review of their role in ocular disease. Clin Sci 131(24):2865–2883
5. Panova IG, Tatikolov AS (2023) Endogenous and exogenous antioxidants as agents preventing the negative effects of contrast media (contrast-induced nephropathy). Pharmaceuticals 16(8):1077
6. Freire VAF, Melo AD, Santos HL, Barros-Pinheiro M (2023) Evaluation of oxidative stress markers in subtypes of preeclampsia: a systematic review and meta-analysis. Placenta 132:55–67
7. Dastogeer KMG, Zahan MI, Rhaman MS, Sarker MSA, Chakraborty A (2022) Microbe-mediated thermotolerance in plants and pertinent mechanisms- a meta-analysis and review. Front Microbiol 13:833566
8. Pei J, Pan X, Wei G, Hua Y (2023) Research progress of glutathione peroxidase family (GPX) in redoxidation. Front Pharmacol 14:1147414
9. Koirala BKS, Moural T, Zhu F (2022) Functional and structural diversity of insect glutathione s-transferases in xenobiotic adaptation. Int J Biol Sci 18(15):5713–5723

10. Park JC, Hagiwara A, Park HG, Lee JS (2020) The glutathione S-transferase genes in marine rotifers and copepods: identification of GSTs and applications for ecotoxicological studies. Mar Pollut Bull 156:111080
11. Gong P, Long H, Guo Y et al (2023) Chinese herbal medicines: the modulator of nonalcoholic fatty liver disease targeting oxidative stress. J Ethnopharmacol 318(Pt B):116927
12. Zhao T, Yang M, Ma L et al (2023) Structural modification and biological activity of polysaccharides. Molecules 28(14):5416
13. Abdul Hakim BN, Xuan NJ, Oslan SNH (2023) A comprehensive review of bioactive compounds from lactic acid bacteria: potential functions as functional food in dietetics and the food industry. Food Secur 12(15):2850
14. Wong SA, Drovandi A, Jones R, Golledge J (2023) Effect of dietary supplements which upregulate nitric oxide on walking and quality of life in patients with peripheral artery disease: a meta-analysis. Biomedicines 11(7):1859
15. Kim MK, Yoon CS, Kim SG, Park YW, Lee SS, Lee SK (2019) Effects of 4-hexylresorcinol on protein expressions in RAW264.7 cells as determined by immunoprecipitation high performance liquid chromatography. Sci Rep 9:3379
16. Yi W, Liu T, Gao X, Xie Y, Liu M (2021) 4-hexylresorcinol inhibits osteoclastogenesis by suppressing the NF-κB signaling pathway and reverses bone loss in ovariectomized mice. Exp Ther Med 21(4):354
17. Liu J, Chen B, Hu Q, Zhang Q, Huang B, Fei P (2023) Pectin grafted with resorcinol and 4-hexylresorcinol: preparation, characterization and application in meat preservation. Int J Biol Macromol 237:124212
18. Pinhal-Enfield G, Ramanathan M, Hasko G et al (2003) An angiogenic switch in macrophages involving synergy between toll-like receptors 2, 4, 7, and 9 and adenosine a(2A) receptors. Am J Pathol 163:711–721
19. Jo YY, Kim DW, Choi JY, Kim SG (2019) 4-hexylresorcinol and silk sericin increase the expression of vascular endothelial growth factor via different pathways. Sci Rep 9:3448
20. Wu WK, Llewellyn OP, Bates DO, Nicholson LB, Dick AD (2010) IL-10 regulation of macrophage VEGF production is dependent on macrophage polarization and hypoxia. Immunobiology 215:796–803
21. Jiménez M, Escribano-Cebrián J, García-Carmona F (1998) Oxidation of the flavonol fisetin by polyphenol oxidase. Biochim Biophys Acta 1425(3):534–542
22. Yen GC, Duh PD, Lin CW (2003) Effects of resveratrol and 4-hexylresorcinol on hydrogen peroxide-induced oxidative DNA damage in human lymphocytes. Free Radic Res 37(5):509–514
23. Murad S (2014) Toll-like receptor 4 in inflammation and angiogenesis: a double-edged sword. Front Immunol 5:313
24. Jo YY, Seo YK, Lee SM, Lee JH, Lee Y, Kim SG (2017) Bone regeneration is associated with the concentration of tumour necrosis factor-α induced by sericin released from a silk mat. Sci Rep 7:15589
25. Albina JE, Mastrofrancesco B, Vessella JA, Louis CA, Henry WL Jr, Reichner JS (2001) HIF-1 expression in healing wounds: HIF-1alpha induction in primary inflammatory cells by TNF-alpha. Am J Physiol Cell Physiol 281:C1971–C1977
26. Haddad JJ, Land SC (2001) A non-hypoxic, ROS sensitive pathway mediates TNF-α-dependent regulation of HIF-1α. FEBS Lett 505:269–274
27. Peyssonnaux C, Datta V, Cramer T et al (2005) HIF-1α expression regulates the bactericidal capacity of phagocytes. J Clin Invest 115(7):1806–1815
28. Bergers G, Brekken R, McMahon G et al (2000) Matrix metalloproteinase-9 triggers the angiogenic switch during carcinogenesis. Nat Cell Biol 2:737–744
29. Wang M, Zhao D, Spinetti G et al (2012) Chronic matrix metalloproteinase inhibition retards age-associated arterial proinflammation and increase in blood pressure. Hypertension 60:459–466

30. Kim DW, Jo YY, Garagiola U et al (2020) Increased level of vascular endothelial growth factors by 4-hexylresorcinol is mediated by transforming growth factor-β1 and accelerates capillary regeneration in the burns in diabetic animals. Int J Mol Sci 21:3473
31. Yamahana H, Terashima M, Takatsuka R et al (2021) TGF-β1 facilitates MT1-MMP-mediated proMMP-9 activation and invasion in oral squamous cell carcinoma cells. Biochem Biophys Rep 27:101072
32. Gomathi K, Rohini M, Vairamani M, Selvamurugan N (2022) Identification and characterization of TGF-β1-responsive Runx2 acetylation sites for matrix metalloproteinase-13 expression in osteoblastic cells. Biochimie 201:1–6
33. Kanokpanonta S, Damrongsakkula S, Ratanavaraporna J, Aramwit P (2013) Physico-chemical properties and efficacy of silk fibroin fabric coated with different waxes as wound dressing. Int J Biol Macromol 55:88–97
34. Baoyong L, Jian Z, Denglong C, Min L (2010) Evaluation of a new type of wound dressing made from recombinant spider silk protein using rat models. Burns 36:891–896
35. Quintana HT, Bortolin JA, da Silva NT, Ribeiro FA, Liberti EA, Ribeiro DA, de Oliveira F (2015) Temporal study following burn injury in young rats is associated with skeletal muscle atrophy, inflammation and altered myogenic regulatory factors. Inflamm Res 64:53–62
36. Moscovis SM, Gordon AE, Al Madani OM et al (2015) Genetic and environmental factors affecting TNF-α responses in relation to sudden infant death syndrome. Front Immunol 6:374
37. Claassen L, Papst S, Reimers K et al (2014) Inflammatory response to burn trauma: nicotine attenuates proinflammatory cytokine levels. Eplasty 14:e46
38. Zhao G, Yu YM, Kaneki M, Bonab AA, Tompkins RG, Fischman AJ (2015) Simvastatin reduces burn injury-induced splenic apoptosis via downregulation of the TNF-α/NF-κB pathway. Ann Surg 261(5):1006–1012
39. Ahn J, Kim SG, Kim MK et al (2016) Topical delivery of 4-hexylresorcinol promotes wound healing via tumor necrosis factor-α suppression. Burns 42:1534–1541
40. Xu F, Zhang C, Graves DT (2013) Abnormal cell responses and role of TNF-α in impaired diabetic wound healing. Biomed Res Int 2013:754802
41. Cholesterol Treatment Trialists' (CTT) Collaboration, Baigent C, Blackwell L et al (2010) Efficacy and safety of more intensive lowering of LDL cholesterol: a meta-analysis of data from 170,000 participants in 26 randomised trials. Lancet 376(9753):1670–1681
42. Thurnher M, Gruenbacher G, Nussbaumer O (2013) Regulation of mevalonate metabolism in cancer and immune cells. Biochim Biophys Acta 1831(6):1009–1015
43. Chiarini A, Petrini P, Bozzini S, Dal Pra I, Armato U (2003) Silk fibroin/poly(carbonate)-urethane as a substrate for cell growth: in vitro interactions with human cells. Biomaterials 24:789–799
44. Łysakowska ME, Ciebiada-Adamiec A, Klimek L, Sienkiewicz M (2015) The activity of silver nanoparticles (Axonnite) on clinical and environmental strains of Acinetobacter spp. Burns 41(2):364–371
45. Boonkaew B, Kempf M, Kimble R, Cuttle L (2014) Cytotoxicity testing of silver-containing burn treatments using primary and immortal skin cells. Burns 40(8):1562–1569
46. Wu J, Zheng Y, Wen X, Lin Q, Chen X, Wu Z (2014) Silver nanoparticle/bacterial cellulose gel membranes for antibacterial wound dressing: investigation in vitro and in vivo. Biomed Mater 9(3):035005
47. Elliott C (2010) The effects of silver dressings on chronic and burns wound healing. Br J Nurs 19(15):S32–S36
48. Wang XQ, Chang HE, Francis R et al (2009) Silver deposits in cutaneous burn scar tissue is a common phenomenon following application of a silver dressing. J Cutan Pathol 36(7):788–792
49. Krishnaraj C, Harper SL, Yun SI (2015) In vivo toxicological assessment of biologically synthesized silver nanoparticles in adult zebrafish (Danio rerio). J Hazard Mater 301:480–491
50. Xu L, Shao A, Zhao Y et al (2015) Neurotoxicity of silver nanoparticles in rat brain after intragastric exposure. J Nanosci Nanotechnol 15(6):4215–4223

51. Kim AS, Chae CH, Kim J, Choi JY, Kim SG, Băciut G (2012) Silver nanoparticles induce apoptosis through the toll-like receptor 2 pathway. Oral Surg Oral Med Oral Pathol Oral Radiol 113(6):789–798
52. Trop M (2006) Silver-coated dressing acticoat caused raised liver enzymes and argyria-like symptoms in burn patient. J Trauma 61(4):1024
53. Evans RT, Baker PJ, Coburn RA, Fischman SL, Genco RJ (1977) In vitro antiplaque effects of antiseptic phenols. J Periodontol 48(3):156–162
54. McNally D, Shephard A, Field E (2012) Randomised, double-blind, placebo-controlled study of a single dose of an amylmetacresol/2,4-dichlorobenzyl alcohol plus lidocaine lozenge or a hexylresorcinol lozenge for the treatment of acute sore throat due to upper respiratory tract infection. J Pharm Pharm Sci 15(2):281–294
55. Iga K, Hussain A, Kashihara T (1981) Effect of complex formation between 4-hexylresorcinol and ethyl myristate on release rate of 4-hexylresorcinol from petrolatum base. J Pharm Sci 70(8):939–943
56. Salla JT, Taddei SR, Queiroz CM, Andrade I Jr, Teixeira MM, Silva TA (2012) The effect of IL-1 receptor antagonist on orthodontic tooth movement in mice. Arch Oral Biol 57:519–524
57. Gostner JM, Becker K, Fuchs D, Sucher R (2013) Redox regulation of the immune response. Redox Rep 18:88–94
58. Shah D, Lynd T, Ho D et al (2020) Pulp–dentin tissue healing response: a discussion of current biomedical approaches. J Clin Med 9:434
59. Sharifi-Rad M, Anil Kumar NV, Zucca P et al (2020) Lifestyle, oxidative stress, and antioxidants: back and forth in the pathophysiology of chronic diseases. Front Physiol 11:694
60. Buczko P, Zalewska A, Szarmach I (2015) Saliva and oxidative stress in oral cavity and in some systemic disorders. J Physiol Pharmacol 66:3–9
61. Leite M, De Lima A, Massuyama M, Otton R (2010) In vivo astaxanthin treatment partially prevents antioxidant alterations in dental pulp from alloxan-induced diabetic rats. Int Endod J 43:959–967
62. Dahiya P, Kamal R, Gupta R, Bhardwaj R, Chaudhary K, Kaur S (2013) Reactive oxygen species in periodontitis. J Indian Soc Periodont 17:411
63. Gate L, Paul J, Ba GN, Tew K, Tapiero H (1999) Oxidative stress induced in pathologies: the role of antioxidants. Biomed Pharmacother 53:169–180
64. Chang JH, Kim DW, Kim SG, Kim TW (2021) Alleviation of oxidative stress in dental pulp cells following 4-hexylresorcinol administration in a rat model. Appl Sci 11:3637
65. Movahed A, Yu L, Thandapilly SJ, Louis XL, Netticadan T (2012) Resveratrol protects adult cardiomyocytes against oxidative stress mediated cell injury. Arch Biochem Biophys 527:74–80
66. Calabrese V, Scuto M, Salinaro AT et al (2020) Hydrogen sulfide and carnosine: modulation of oxidative stress and inflammation in kidney and brain axis. Antioxidants 9:1303
67. Cooper PR, Holder MJ, Smith AJ (2014) Inflammation and regeneration in the dentin-pulp complex: a double-edged sword. J Endod 40:S46–S51
68. Diomede F, Marconi GD, Guarnieri S et al (2020) A novel role of ascorbic acid in anti-inflammatory pathway and ROS generation in HEMA treated dental pulp stem cells. Materials 13:130
69. Okabe E (1994) Endogenous vasoactive substances and oxygen-derived free radicals in pulpal haemodynamics. Arch Oral Biol 39:S39–S45
70. Viduskalne I, Care R (2010) Analysis of the crown fractures and factors affecting pulp survival due to dental trauma. Stomatologija 12:109–115
71. Ozçelik B, Kuraner T, Kendir B, Aşan E (2000) Histopathological evaluation of the dental pulps in crown-fractured teeth. J Endod 26:271–273
72. Ighodaro O, Akinloye O (2017) First line defence antioxidants-superoxide dismutase (SOD), catalase (CAT) and glutathione peroxidase (GPX): their fundamental role in the entire antioxidant defence grid. Alexandria J Med 54:287–293

73. Xiong W, Ma H, Zhang Z et al (2020) The protective effect of icariin and phosphorylated icariin against LPS-induced intestinal goblet cell dysfunction. Innate Immun 26:97–106
74. Topçu KÇ, Kırıcı D, Evcil M (2016) Catalase activity in healthy and inflamed pulp tissues of permanent teeth in young people. Niger J Clin Pract 19:600–602
75. Bagheri A, Ebrahimpour S, Nourbakhsh N, Talebi S, Esmaeili A (2021) Protective effect of quercetin on alteration of antioxidant genes expression and histological changes in the dental pulp of the streptozotocin-diabetic rats. Arch Oral Biol 125:105088
76. Kim JH, Kim DW, Kim SG, Kim TW (2020) 4-hexylresorcinol administration increases dental hard tissue formation and incisor eruption rate in rats. Appl Sci 10:5511

Chapter 5
4-Hexylresorcinol as Histone Deacetylase Inhibitor

Abstract This chapter investigates the role of 4-hexylresorcinol (4HR) as a histone deacetylase inhibitor (HDACi) specifically targeting Class I and IIa HDACs and its potential therapeutic applications. While 4HR does not directly inhibit Class III HDACs (sirtuins), it has been observed to impact the expression of SIRT3 and 6 through other mechanisms, such as modulating NAD+ levels. The chapter also delves into the effects of 4HR on growing animals, emphasizing the gender-specific influences on body weight, mandibular size, and hormonal levels. These findings underscore the complex relationship between 4HR, its HDACi activity, and hormonal regulation. Further research is needed to better understand the mechanisms behind these effects and to explore the full therapeutic potential of 4HR as an HDACi.

Keywords 4-hexylresorcinol (4HR) · Histone deacetylase inhibitor · Sirtuin · Gender-specific effects · Mandibular size · Body weight

The acetyl group is an important functional residue, and acetylation and deacetylation are processes that regulate the function of proteins. Histone deacetylase (HDAC) is an enzyme that removes acetyl groups from lysine, which is an amino acid that is present in many types of proteins [1]. This posttranslational modification of proteins, which involves adding or removing the acetyl group from lysine, has a significant impact on the conformation and function of the proteins [2].

DNA has a strong negative charge due to the presence of phosphate groups. Histone, on the other hand, has a positive charge and provides binding to DNA. Acetylation of histone causes it to lose its positive charge, thus relaxing the binding between histone and DNA. This relaxation allows many proteins involved in DNA transcription to bind to the promoter region of the target gene, thus regulating specific gene transcription [1, 2]. In addition to histone, the functions of other proteins are influenced by HDACs during the posttranslational modification process [2]. HDACs can be classified into four groups (Table 5.1) and can be found in various intracellular locations depending on their functional requirements, with the nucleus and mitochondria being the main localizations [1].

S.-G. Kim, *Biomedical Application of 4-Hexylresorcinol*,
https://doi.org/10.1007/978-981-97-0637-2_5

Table 5.1 Classification of HDAC

Class	Members
I	HDAC1, 2, 3, 8
IIA	HDAC4, 5, 7, 9
IIB	HDAC6, 10
III	SIRT1, 2, 3, 4, 5, 6, 7
IV	HDAC11

HDAC histone deacetylase, *SIRT* sirtuin

Class I HDACs have been found to be involved in a wide range of physiological processes and diseases, such as cardiovascular disease, auto-immune disease, musculoskeletal disease, and malignancy [3]. HDAC1 is known to regulate gene expression, and its expression is increased in transformed cells [4]. HDAC2 is overexpressed in pancreatic cancer [5] and pathologic cardiomegaly [6]. The administration of HDACi (HDAC Inhibitors) such as trichostatin A (TSA) is known to be effective in treating cardiac hypertrophy [7, 8]. TSA has also been used for the treatment of rheumatism by suppressing the expression level of tumor necrosis factor-α (TNF-α) and interleukin-6 (IL-6) [9]. In addition, the administration of butyrate, a bacterial-derived organic chemical with HDACi activity, has been found to reduce pain in epileptic rats [10] and inhibit the proliferation of colorectal cancer cells [11]. Valproic acid, originally developed as an anti-convulsant, has been identified as an HDACi and has been found to improve nerve regeneration and motor function in a damaged rat model [12]. Collectively, these findings suggest that HDAC inhibitors may be promising therapeutic agents for a variety of diseases.

Resorcinolic lipids are organic chemicals of plant and bacterial origin [13]. 4-Hexylresorcinol (4HR) is a synthetic resorcinolic lipid developed as an antiseptic agent [13]. It has been found to suppress the respiration of microorganisms and induce dormancy [14], as well as bind to tyrosinase and inhibit its activity, thereby preventing melanosis of food [15]. To assess its safety as a food additive, toxicological studies have been conducted, and anticancer effects have been observed [16, 17]. Subsequently, the anticancer mechanisms of 4HR have been investigated in greater detail [18, 19]. Studies have shown that 4HR suppresses the nuclear factor-κB (NF-κB) pathway in oral cancer cells by inhibiting transglutaminase-2 (TG-2) [18, 20]. Additionally, 4HR administration has been found to reduce the formation of foreign body giant cells in the silk-based graft material [21] and suppress TNF-α expression in a deep burn [22].

Recently, 4HR has been identified as potent M2 macrophages polarizing agent [23]. Studies have demonstrated that 4HR increases transforming growth factor-β1 (TGF-β1) expression while decreasing TNF-α expression in RAW263.7 cells [24]. In addition, 4HR has also been shown to increase the expression level of vascular endothelial cell growth factor (VEGF) via TGF-β1-mediated pathway in human umbilical endothelial cells (HUVECs) [25].

Upon further investigation into the mechanism of TGF-β1 expression by 4HR administration, it was found that the broad function of 4HR bears resemblance to that of other histone deacetylase inhibitors (HDACi). This similarity can be attributed to the presence of a hydrophobic alkyl group in 4HR [13], with a length like that of the functional group in other HDACi [26]. In addition, despite the absence of an acetyl group at the end of the hexyl group in 4HR, the hydroxyl-benzene can act as a cap group.

5.1 4HR Inhibits Class I and IIa HDAC Activity

New studies have uncovered the multifaceted effects of 4HR, including antimicrobial, anticancer, proangiogenic, anti-inflammatory, and metabolic effects, which suggest its broad-spectrum regulation of cellular events. Posttranslational modifications, such as those mediated by HDACs, are crucial for the epigenetic regulation of various cellular processes [3]. Interestingly, our latest research found that 4HR can decrease the expression of Class I and IIa HDACs in HUVECs [27]. Moreover, 4HR was observed to inhibit the enzymatic activity of Class I HDACs and increase the levels of acetylated proteins [27]. It is noteworthy that the pattern of HDAC inhibition by 4HR is like that of TSA, a well-known HDAC inhibitor, at different doses [27].

The hydrophobic pocket of each HDAC constitutes its enzymatic domain, and the length of this pocket may vary depending on the type of HDAC (Fig. 5.1). 4HR has a

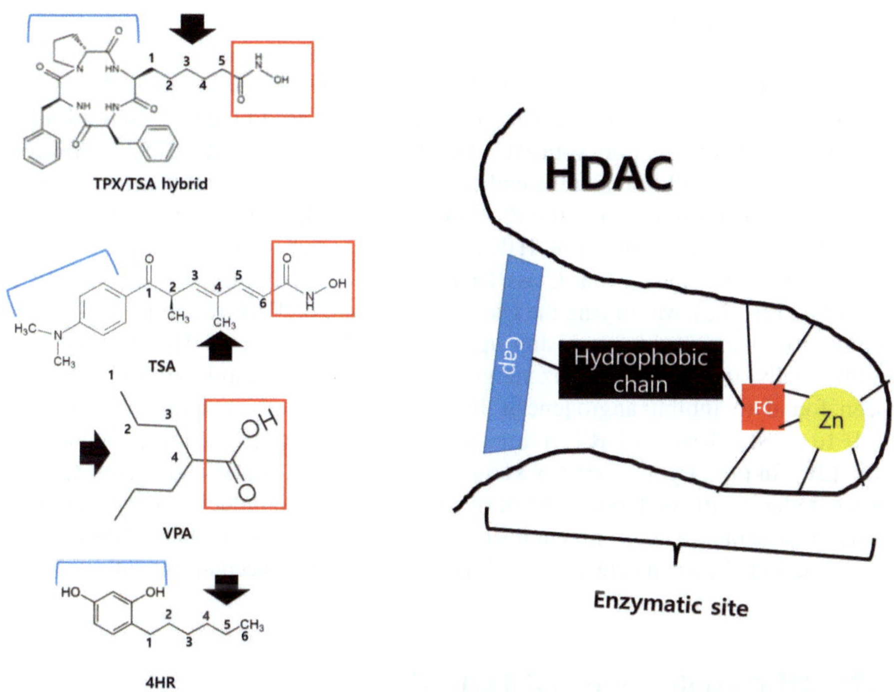

Fig. 5.1 HDAC inhibitors (HDACi) contain a hydrophobic group, functional group, and a cap, which interact with zinc ions and the surrounding amino acids to form hydrogen bonds. Examples of HDACi include trapoxin (TPX), trichostatin A (TSA) hybrid, TSA, and valproic acid (VPA). 4HR has a cap and hydrophobic chain; if positioned in the opposite direction, the hydroxyl groups can act as a functional group, chelating the zinc ions

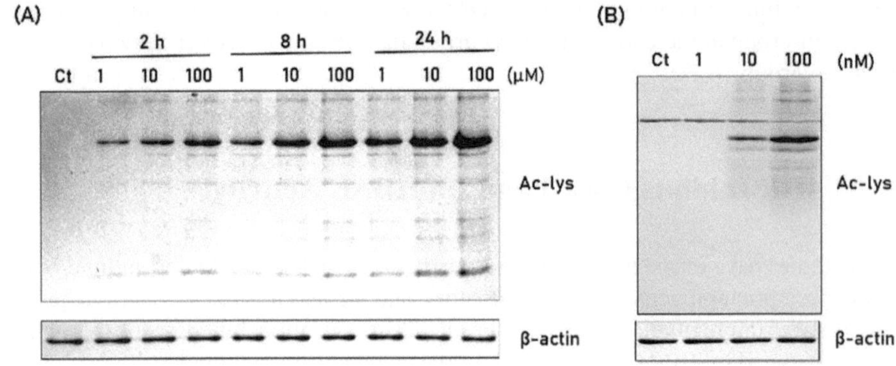

Fig. 5.2 The expression level of acetylated proteins in whole cellular lysates of human umbilical vein endothelial cells was found to be increased following treatment with either 4HR (**a**) or TSA (**b**). This indicates that both 4HR (**a**) and TSA (**b**) administration can effectively induce acetylation of proteins in these cells (modified from author's previous publication [27])

six-carbon alkyl group that gives it a high degree of hydrophobicity [13]. This length of hydrophobic domain is comparable to other known HDAC inhibitors, suggesting that 4HR may act as a decoy molecule that can block the hydrophobic enzymatic domain (Fig. 5.1). TSA is a known HDAC inhibitor with the same number of carbon chains as 4HR (Fig. 5.1), and its derivatives have a similar structure [28]. Thus, 4HR may be able to competitively inhibit HDACs in a similar way to TSA and its derivatives.

The expression level of acetylated proteins is increased by either 4HR administration or TSA administration in HUVEC (Fig. 5.2). Compared to TSA, 4HR does not possess an acetyl group at the end of its alkyl chain, which could affect its binding affinity to HDACs. While the IC50 of TSA on HDAC has been measured to be <38 nM [26], the exact IC50 of 4HR on HDAC has yet to be determined. Cellular experiments have shown that Class I HDAC activity is inhibited at 1 μM 4HR in HUVEC (Fig. 5.2). Modifying the chemical structure of 4HR by adding an acetyl or amine group may be a promising approach to develop novel HDAC inhibitors. Additionally, the hydroxyl-benzene group could act as a cap (Fig. 5.1). TSA has been found to inhibit angiogenesis by suppressing hypoxia inducible factor-1α (HIF1α) [28], whereas 4HR increases angiogenesis via a HIF1α-independent pathway [29]. In prokaryotes, 4HR is known to act as an antiseptic and chemical chaperone, reducing the metabolic rate of microorganisms and inducing a dormant state, which is resistant to environmental stress [13, 14]. It is possible that 4HR may have similar effects in eukaryotes, although further research is needed to confirm this.

5.2 4HR Application and TGF-β1

In a previous study, we investigated the effects of 4HR on human umbilical vein endothelial cells (HUVEC) and found that it could enhance vascular endothelial growth factor (VEGF) expression through a pathway independent of HIF [29]. We also observed that 4HR-induced apoptotic stress could increase the expression of transforming growth factor-β1 (TGF-β1) [25]. Further experiments showed that siRNA targeting TGF-β1 could reduce the expression of VEGF in HUVEC, whereas TGF-β1-induced angiogenesis could increase capillary formation in a diabetic animal model [25]. Interestingly, supplementing TGF-β1 with VEGF resulted in early wound closure and improved angiogenesis and vasculogenesis [30]. Additionally, we found that treating stem cells with TGF-β1 induced cellular differentiation into functional pericyte-like cells [31].

Cellular stress has been shown to be transmitted to both the mitochondria and the endoplasmic reticulum (ER), leading to physiological or pathological events [32]. These stressed organelles are known to play a role in cellular differentiation and apoptosis [32]. When the mitochondria and the ER fail to maintain homeostasis, apoptosis can be triggered (Fig. 5.3). On the other hand, successful adaptation of the cell can lead to cellular growth and differentiation. An increase in ER stress has been found to be linked to increased expression of the cytokine TGF-β1 [33]. This suggests that increased levels of TGF-β1 in endothelial cells may be due to ER stress-induced differentiation. Tauroursodeoxycholate (TUDCA) has been used to relieve ER stress [34]. Therefore, the effects of 4HR administration on ER stress can be evaluated by measuring the changes in TGF-β1 expression with and without

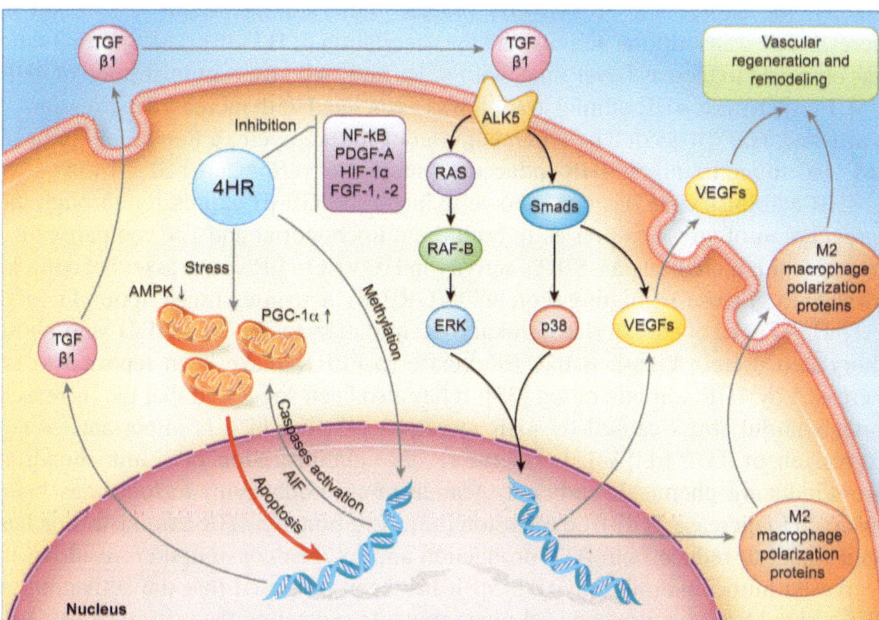

Fig. 5.3 The schematic drawing for the proposed mechanism indicates that apoptotic stress on the mitochondria is induced by application of 4HR, which subsequently induces TGF-β1 expression. The secreted TGF-β1 protein then binds to ALK5 and initiates a downstream signal through the RAS/Smads pathway, resulting in increased expression of VEGFs (reproduced from author's previous publication [36])

TUDCA addition. In fact, the addition of TUDCA has been found to attenuate 4HR-induced TGF-β1 expression [35].

Numerous proteins participate in the response of ER and mitochondria to cellular stress. One group of proteins that has garnered considerable attention is the sirtuins (SIRTs), which belong to the class III HDACs and are comprised of seven distinct isoforms (SIRT1–7) [37]. These enzymes are predominantly located in the nucleus and mitochondria, and their expression levels are upregulated in response to cellular stress, aiding cells in maintaining homeostasis [32, 38].

4HR is a compound that has been shown to induce several antioxidant proteins in RAW 264.7 cells [24] and human umbilical vein endothelial cells (HUVECs) [36] and to have similar antioxidant activity to resveratrol in HUVECs [29] and lymphocytes [39]. As SIRTs are known to induce antioxidant enzymes, it is possible that 4HR may also act as an SIRT activator, thereby reducing mitochondrial and ER stress. Additionally, inhibition of specificity protein 1 (Sp1) disrupts ER homeostasis [40], and 4HR has been demonstrated to increase Sp1 expression in SCC-9 cells (tongue cancer cells) and induce cellular differentiation [19]. These findings suggest that 4HR may have a role in modulating the adaptive response of the ER and mitochondria to cellular stress.

It has long been established that hyperacetylation of histone 3 (H3) is essential for the expression of TGF-β1 [41]. Class I HDACs are known to be inhibited by 4HR [27], which has been shown to induce hyperacetylation of H3, and consequently, the expression of TGF-β1. In fact, 4HR administration was found to increase Sp1 transcription activity and the acetylation of H3 [35]. The Sp1/Sp3 ratio was observed to increase over time, with 8, 16, and 24 h post-administration of 4HR [35]. Furthermore, 4HR administration was associated with increased expression of p-Sp1 and TGF-β1 [35]. The administration of mithramycin, a known inhibitor of Sp1, was found to inhibit 4HR-induced expression of p-Sp1 and TGF-β1 [35].

4HR administration has been shown to increase TGF-β1 expression through the upregulation of stress responses in both the mitochondrial and ER compartments, together with increased pan-SIRTs activity in HUVECs. ER stress-associated markers such as glucose-regulating protein 78 (GRP78), activating transcription factor 4 (ATF4), ATF6α, phosphorylated eukaryotic initiation factor 2 (p-eIF2), and phosphorylated protein kinase R-like ER kinase (p-PERK) have been reported to be increased by 4HR administration [35]. It has also been suggested that the increased mitochondrial stress caused by 4HR increases p-Sp1, which is important for the expression of TGF-β1 [42]. Furthermore, the administration of a mitochondrial stress-inducing chemical, carbonyl cyanide m-chlorophenylhydrazone, has been observed to increase TGF-β1 expression [43]. Additionally, 4HR administration has been found to reduce both ATP production and oxygen consumption, resulting in decreased mitochondrial activity [35]. It has been proposed that the activation of SIRTs should favor mitochondrial function while protecting them from stress [44], and it has been observed that 4HR increases SIRT6 expression and pan-SIRTs activity as a delayed response [35]. The increased mitochondrial membrane potential at 24 h after 4HR administration may be due to the protective activity of SIRTs [35], and it has been observed that hyper-acetylated H3 is also required for the expression of TGF-β1, with this response being enhanced by HDACi [41]. In fact, H3 has been reported to be hyper-acetylated by 4HR administration [35].

It has been suggested that 4HR exhibits a wide variety of functions, such as anti-cancer effects [19], anti-browning effects [45], anti-inflammatory effects [22], and increased bone formation [21]. These divergent effects are likely to be involved in the broad-spectrum regulation of cellular events [23, 46], and it has been proposed that 4HR increases TGF-β1 expression via hyper-acetylated H3 and p-Sp1 (Fig. 5.4).

When cells experience ER stress, the machinery for restoring ER homeostasis is activated [29]. This is achieved by reducing active protein synthesis and increasing the expression of chaperones [47, 48]. Additionally, organic chemicals can induce ER stress by binding to intracellular decoy proteins and changing protein conformation, leading to the production of misfolded proteins [49]. To counteract this, the transcription factor ATF6 is activated, leading to the removal of misfolded proteins [50]. 4HR administration increases the expression level of ATF6α, as well as the expression levels of p–PERK, p-eIF2, and ATF4 [35], which reduce protein

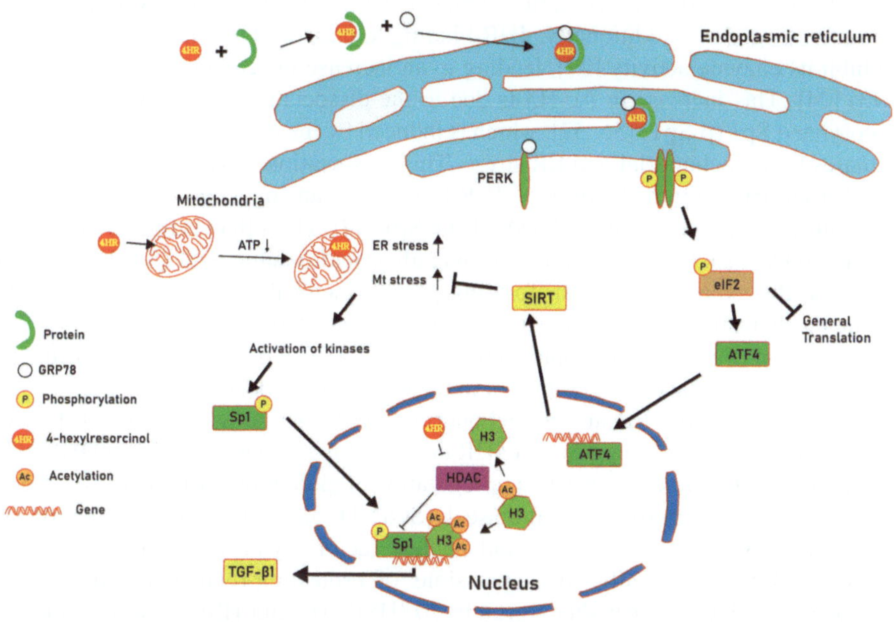

Fig. 5.4 A schematic drawing of the signaling pathway involved in 4HR administration-induced mitochondrial and endoplasmic reticulum (ER) stress has been presented. It has been demonstrated that ER stress-induced activating transcription factor 4 (ATF4) expression increases sirtuin (SIRT) activity, which in turn alleviates mitochondrial stress and kinases activation. Moreover, mitochondrial stress is known to increase the phosphorylation of Sp1, which is essential for the activation of the transcription factor transforming growth factor-β1 (TGF-β1). However, for the activation of TGF-β1 transcription, not only p-Sp1 but also hyper-acetylated histone H3 is required. Since 4HR is a class I histone deacetylase (HDAC) inhibitor, it reduces the expression levels of HDAC4 and HDAC5, thus allowing H3 to be hyper-acetylated by 4HR administration (reproduced from author's previous publication [35])

translation activity [51]. Administration of the ER stress inhibitor TUDCA decreased the expression of ER stress markers such as ATF6α, p–PERK, p-eIF2, and ATF4, which were increased by 4HR administration [35]. Additionally, TUDCA decreased 4HR-induced TGF-β1 expression, which is known to increase VEGF expression in HUVECs and help differentiate HUVECs [25, 35].

The administration of 4HR on human umbilical vein endothelial cells (HUVECs) induces ER stress [35]. This is likely due to the long alkyl group of 4HR, which can bind to any hydrophobic domain of proteins with varying affinity [52]. Chromatography with 4HR-bound beads has confirmed that some proteins show high affinity for 4HR, leading to a change in protein conformation and thus the formation of misfolded proteins [24]. The misfolded proteins are then recognized by the binding protein GRP78, which transports them to the ER [53]. This protein complex then phosphorylates the PERK protein and activates the transcription factor ATF4, subsequently leading to an increase in apoptotic stress [35].

The administration of 4HR has been shown to reduce ATP synthesis in mitochondria [35] and increase NAD+ levels [54]. This increased NAD+ level has been found to increase SIRT transcription [55], which is further increased by 4HR administration (Fig. 5.4). Additionally, 4HR binding to class I HDAC has been shown to inhibit its enzyme activity [27], leading to an increase in acetylated histone 3 (Ac-H3) [24]. This increase in Ac-H3 is due to the dissociation of HDAC from phosphorylated Sp1 (p-Sp1) [56, 57], which is induced by the phosphorylation of several kinases by mitochondrial and ER stress. This dissociation of HDAC from p-Sp1 is further increased by the binding of 4HR to HDAC, causing a conformation change and subsequent dissociation of HDAC from Sp1 [42]. This effect is further enhanced using HDACi such as TSA and suberoylanilide hydroxamic acid (SAHA), which increase the expression of transforming growth factor-β1 (TGF-β1) through this same mechanism [42]. These events, when activated, lead to an increase in TGF-β1 transcription (Fig. 5.3). The topical application of 4HR has also been demonstrated to accelerate capillary regeneration in diabetic animal models [25].

The results of the ER and mitochondrial stress tests, as well as the IP-HPLC experiments (Fig. 5.5), suggest that 4HR has a potent antioxidant effect in HUVECs [35]. The results showed consistent upregulation of glutathione S-transferase omega 1 (GSTO1) and superoxide dismutase-1 (SOD-1), as well as downregulation of nitric oxide synthase-1 (NOS-1) and nuclear factor erythroid 2–related factor 2 (NRF2) [35]. Additionally, the expressions of protection-related proteins heme-oxygenase 1 (HO-1), heat shock protein-70 (HSP-70), and HSP-90 were found to be simultaneously downregulated (Fig. 5.5). These results suggest that the local administration of 4HR may be safe in the absence of oxidative cellular damage.

4HR is a potent antiseptic agent that is known to kill actively proliferating microorganisms [58]. This antiseptic action of 4HR can be considered as a form of stress on the microorganism. However, some microorganisms have been found to reduce their metabolic rate and enter a state of dormancy after the administration of 4HR [14]. This suggests that 4HR may act as a chemical chaperone, due to its amphiphilic structure, like other chemical chaperones [13]. Microorganisms in a state of dormancy are known to be more resistant to environmental stress [14], indicating that

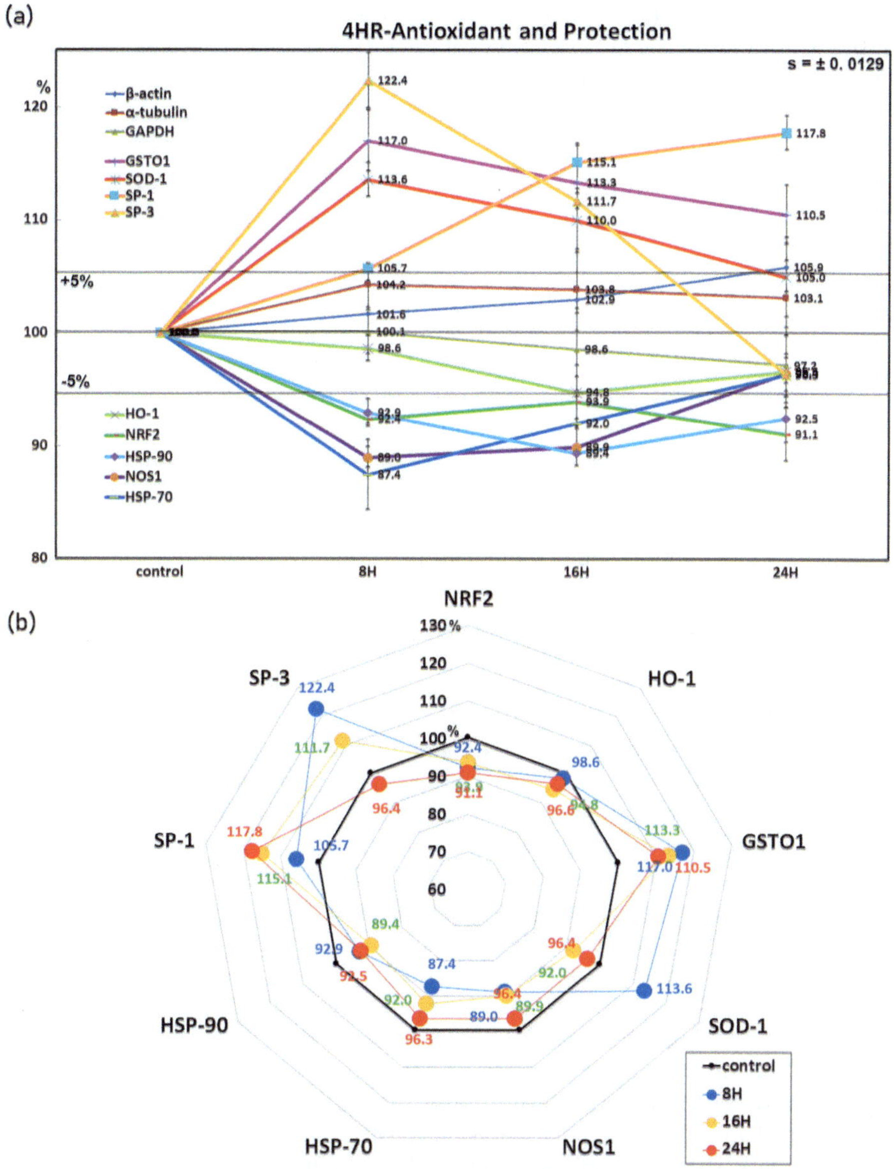

Fig. 5.5 IP-HPLC analysis. The expression of antioxidant- and protection-related proteins in 4HR-treated HUVECs was investigated. Results showed that the antioxidant proteins GSTO1 and SOD-1 were upregulated by 4HR compared to the untreated control, while the antioxidant regulating transcription factor NRF2 and protection-related proteins HO-1, HSP-70, and HSP-90 were downregulated. Additionally, Sp-1 expression was gradually increased by 5.7%, 15.1%, and 17.8% at 8, 16, and 24 h, respectively, while Sp-3 expression was increased up to 122.4% at 8 h but gradually decreased to normal level at 24 h. These results were illustrated in a line graph (**a**) and a star plot (**b**), which showed the protein expression (%) at 8, 16, or 24 h after 4HR administration, and the differential expression levels (%) respectively (reproduced from author's own study [35])

4HR may be mimicking its action in prokaryotes in eukaryotes as well. However, further studies are needed to clarify the differences in detail between the two chemicals. Tauroursodeoxycholic acid (TUDCA) is another chemical chaperone that has an amphiphilic structure, like 4HR [34]. However, unlike 4HR, TUDCA is known to alleviate ER stress [34]. The difference in chemical structure between the two chemicals may explain why they have different cellular responses after administration.

5.3 4HR Application and SIRTs

Fresh research has indicated that yeast contains prototype SIRTs, which appear to be associated with extended lifespan [59]. Interestingly, it has been observed that when cellular metabolism is restricted, the expression of SIRT1 is upregulated in muscle cells [60]. SIRT3, on the other hand, is predominantly expressed in mitochondria and plays a crucial role in energy metabolism [61], while SIRT6 appears to inhibit glucose uptake and metabolism [62]. Moreover, administering 4HR has been shown to increase the expression of both SIRT3 and SIRT6 in Saos-2 cells [54]. Our recent study found that administering 4HR to HUVEC resulted in decreased mitochondrial respiratory activity and ATP synthesis [35]. These findings suggest that inhibition of mitochondrial activity by 4HR could be linked to an increase in SIRT3 and SIRT6 expression.

It has been demonstrated that 4HR administration can reduce mitochondrial activity and may be fatal to cancer cells. Studies have also revealed that 4HR administration has anticancer activity, which can inhibit the growth of tumors [63, 64]. However, cancer cells that survive 4HR treatment may be more resistant to other cancer therapies due to increased levels of SIRT3 and SIRT6, which can play a protective role [29, 65]. Thus, further research is needed to understand the role of SOD activation and SIRT3/SIRT6 in 4HR-mediated cancer cell survival.

It has been observed that 4HR administration increases the expression level of SIRT6 [54] (Fig. 5.6). SIRT6 is known to reduce inflammation and fatty liver formation induced by a high-fat diet [66]. SIRT6 reduces aging-associated inflammatory reactions by inhibiting the nuclear factor kappa B (NF-κB) pathway [67]. Additionally, 4HR has been shown to be a strong inhibitor of the NF-κB pathway [46, 68] and to reduce the expression of NF-κB while increasing IκB kinase in HUVECs [36]. These findings suggest that 4HR administration may be a promising therapeutic avenue for the treatment of inflammatory diseases.

New research has indicated that the activity of SIRTs is highly dependent on the level of NAD+ present in cells [69]. Interestingly, when nutrients are scarce, AMP-activated protein kinase (AMPK) is activated, resulting in an increase in NAD+ levels [69]. Furthermore, when fibroblast growth factor 21 (FGF21) is administered, it has been found to activate SIRT1, which is linked to reductions in body weight [70]. Additionally, SIRT activity can be modulated by changes in the levels of NAD+ [71]. NAD+ is also used by poly (ADP-ribose) polymerases (PARPs) and

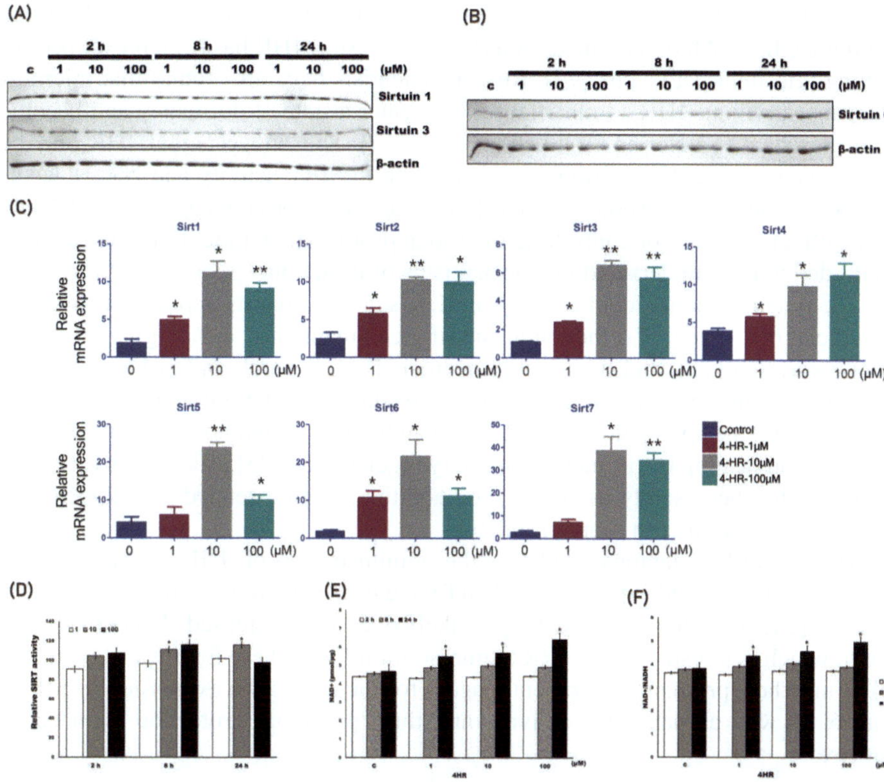

Fig. 5.6 The administration of 4HR had a significant effect on the expression and activity of SIRT enzymes in HUVECs. The expression level of SIRT1 and 3 was not significantly changed by 4HR administration (**a**). However, the expression level of SIRT6 was increased by 4HR administration (**b**). Quantitative RT-PCR results showed that the expression of SIRT1 and 3 did not change, while the expression of SIRT6 was significantly increased (**c**) ($*P < 0.05$, $**P < 0.01$ compared to untreated control). Moreover, the administration of 4HR (1–100 μM) increased pan-SIRTs enzyme activity (**d**) ($*P < 0.05$ compared to the control group). Additionally, 4HR increased NAD+ production (**e**) ($*P < 0.05$ compared to the control group) and the NAD+ to NADH ratio (**f**). These results indicate that 4HR administration has a positive effect on SIRT expression and activity in HUVECs (modified from author' publication [54])

cyclic ADP-ribose synthases as an enzyme substrate [55]. Since PARPs are DNA repair enzymes and are highly expressed in cancer cells, inhibiting them could be beneficial for cancer treatment [72]. The inhibition of PARPs may result in the flooding of NAD+ and lead to SIRT activation. Although the administration of 4HR has been shown to increase NAD+ levels and the NAD+/NADH ratio [54], its effect on PARPs is still not fully understood. Further research is required to explore the connection between PARPs and the administration of 4HR.

Recent studies have demonstrated that derivatives of resorcinolic lipids can suppress microbial proliferation, and the application of 4HR has been shown to be an effective inhibitor of microbial growth [13]. However, when 4HR is administered orally, its absorption rate from the gastrointestinal tract is rather poor [52]. In fact, studies have indicated that only 18% of the initial dosage is found in the urine within the first 12 h of administration [52]. As a result, 4HR has been prescribed for killing intestinal pathogens [73]. Russian scientists have also found that microorganisms surviving 4HR administration may enter a state of dormancy and become more resistant to outer environmental stress [14]. This suggests that 4HR may be acting as a chemical chaperone, as an increase in SIRT activity and NAD+ levels has been observed in response to 4HR [14]. Thus, it can be concluded that 4HR may be an effective agent for controlling microbial proliferation, though further research is needed to fully understand the mechanisms of its action.

The potential antioxidant activity of 4HR suggests that its applications may be beneficial in a variety of orthodontic and surgical treatments, such as gingivitis [74], root resorption [75], and dental pulp necrosis [76]. Several studies have reported that antioxidant activity can affect the manifestation of these conditions [24, 29]. Furthermore, the application of 4HR ointment has been found to accelerate diabetic burn wound healing by promoting capillary regeneration [25]. Additionally, the fact that 4HR has been safely used as a food additive for an extended period [52] may make its utilization even more promising.

This study has demonstrated that the administration of 4HR on Saos-2 cells results in an increased expression of SIRT3 and 6, as well as an increased pan-SIRT activity [54]. This increase in activity is likely due to the increased NAD+ to NADH ratio, which is a result of the 4HR administration [54]. These findings suggest that 4HR may be a promising therapeutic agent for increasing the expression of SIRT3 and 6, as well as pan-SIRT activity, and thus, providing protection from cellular stress.

5.4 The Application of 4HR in Growing Animal

It has been suggested that the broad spectrum of HDAC activity may influence skeletal development [77–79]. Studies have demonstrated that systemic administration of HDACi, such as valproate, can reduce bone mineral density in children [77]. In addition, a study of 4HR showed HDACi activity on osteoblast-like cells (Saos-2 cells) [80]. Interestingly, the systemic administration of 4HR had a different effect on males and females, which was closely associated with the serum testosterone level [80]. This was evidenced by the fact that 4HR-administered young male rats showed a relatively smaller size of the mandible (Fig. 5.7).

Even though 4HR has been used as a food additive [81], the safety of its chronic administration has been called into question [82]. Nevertheless, a study on ovariectomized rat models has revealed that 4HR administration does not have any oestrogen-like effect [83]. Furthermore, when 4HR was administered to 4-week-old female rats for a period of 3 months, the serum levels of oestrogen did not differ significantly from those of the untreated control group [80].

The results of a study examining the effects of 4HR administration on body weight and mandibular size in male and female rats showed that 4HR administration did not significantly affect female body weight [80]. However, male rats treated with 4HR administration showed a delay in body weight increase, approximately a week behind the control group [80]. Additionally, the serum level of testosterone in the 4HR-treated young male rat group was significantly lower than that of the untreated control group ($p < 0.05$) [80]. This decrease in testosterone levels due to 4HR administration was correlated with a decrease in mandibular size [80]. In contrast, the administration of anabolic steroids in 5-week-old female rats resulted in an increase in body weight and skull length [84]. This suggests that the reduction in testosterone levels due to 4HR administration has a different effect on body weight and mandibular size in male and female rats. Furthermore, the single-nucleotide polymorphism of aromatase was found to have a significant effect on mandibular growth only in human boys, not girls [85]. This further supports the idea that the effects of 4HR administration on body weight and mandibular size are gender-specific.

Recent studies have suggested a relationship between HDACi and testosterone levels. Valproic acid, an antiepileptic drug, has been demonstrated to possess HDACi activity, and its administration in male mice has been shown to reduce serum testosterone levels [86]. Conversely, valproic acid administration on cultured porcine ovarian follicular cells has been observed to increase testosterone secretion [87]. This suggests that the effect of valproic acid administration may differ depending on the administration method and animal model [86]. Additionally, a single injection of valproic acid in new-born mice has been reported to increase the acetylation level of H3 [87], and 4-h administration of valproic acid has been observed to increase H3 acetylation in Saos-2 cells [80]. Furthermore, reduced steroid hormone levels due to valproic acid administration have been suggested to be mediated by mitochondrial stress [88]. Additionally, sodium butyrate, another HDACi, has been observed to eliminate the effect of testosterone on C. elegans behavior when

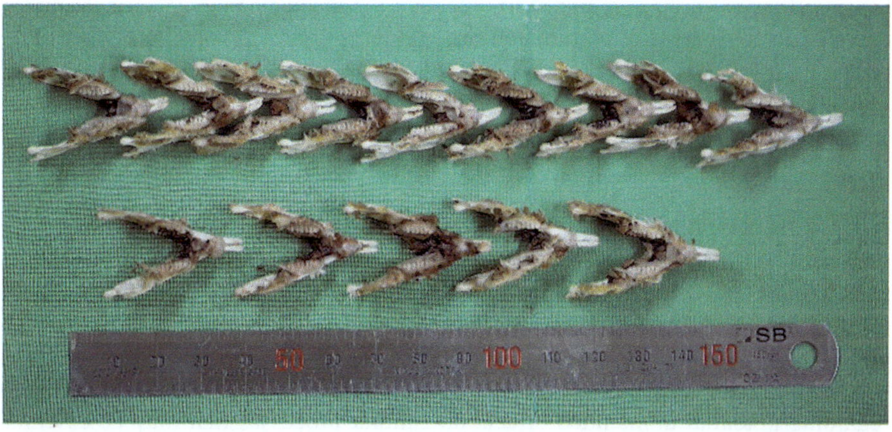

Fig. 5.7 The results of the comparison of mandible size between 4HR-treated and untreated control groups revealed that the size of the mandible was significantly smaller in the 4HR-treated group compared to the untreated control group (Data from the author's previous study [80])

administered acutely [89]. These findings suggest that there may be a similar mechanism between 4HR and valproic acid in steroid-hormone-associated cellular response, which should be further investigated.

Patients with hypoparathyroidism have been found to have decreased mandibular cortical thickness [90]. Sanjad-Sakati syndrome, a rare genetic disorder, is strongly associated with hypoparathyroidism and micrognathia [91]. In a study of young male rats, the 4HR treatment group showed small mandibles and decreased parathyroid hormone (PTH) levels [80]. While PTH has been found to regulate HDAC4 in UMR 106–01 cells [92], the exact mechanism between HDACi and PTH expression has yet to be determined. Additionally, noggin, an inhibitory protein of bone morphogenic protein-4 (BMP-4), has been linked to small mandibles through its polymorphism [93]. The serum level of BMP-4 was found to be increased in the 4HR-treated young male rat group [80].

It has been observed that 4HR treatment of young female rat results in an increase in mandibular size, as opposed to male rats, which do not demonstrate such an effect [80]. This phenomenon is likely attributed to the elevated growth hormone (GH) and growth hormone-releasing hormone (GHRH) levels observed in the 4HR-treated young female group, which are not present in the 4HR-treated young male group [80]. This is supported by the finding that GH deficiency results in small mandibles [94], and exogenous GH administration can improve body weight and growth in rats that are small for gestational age [95]. Additionally, the administration of TSA, an inhibitor of HDACi, increases GH-mRNA expression level in pituitary cells [96]. However, the 4HR administration appears to reduce testosterone levels in both young male and female groups [80], but the effect of this reduction in the female group may not have been strong enough to induce a significant effect on skeletal development, as the baseline testosterone levels in female rats are already relatively low. Thus, it is likely that the elevated expression of GH and GHRH in the 4HR-treated young female group is what induced the observed mandibular growth [80]. Further research is required to elucidate the mechanism of the sexual differences in response to 4HR administration.

5.5 Closing Remark

Acetylation and deacetylation are essential processes in cellular signalling pathways that can affect many cellular events. The modulation of these processes has been identified as a potential therapeutic strategy for various diseases. HDAC inhibitors such as 4HR have shown promise in preclinical and clinical studies for their ability to alter gene expression and protein function via the modulation of acetylation levels. However, the broad range of actions of HDAC inhibitors raises concerns regarding potential unintended effects on cellular processes that may be essential for normal cellular function.

As such, before the administration of HDAC inhibitors such as 4HR, it is important to carefully evaluate the potential benefits and risks on a case-by-case basis.

Additionally, preclinical and clinical studies should be conducted to elucidate the specific mechanisms and targets of HDAC inhibitors to better understand their potential therapeutic benefits and risks. By carefully considering the indications for HDAC inhibitor administration and conducting further research, we can maximize the therapeutic potential of these drugs while minimizing their potential unintended consequences.

References

1. Haberland M, Montgomery RL, Olson EN (2009) The many roles of histone deacetylases in development and physiology: implications for disease and therapy. Nat Rev Genet 10:32–42
2. Aka JA, Kim GW, Yang XJ (2011) In: Yao-Seto (ed) Histone deacetylases: the biology and clinical implication. Springer, New York, NY, pp 1–12; ISBN 978-3-642-21630-5
3. Reichert N, Choukrallah MA, Matthias P (2012) Multiple roles of class I HDACs in proliferation, differentiation, and development. Cell Mol Life Sci 69:2173–2187
4. Bartl S, Taplick J, Lagger G, Khier H, Kuchler K, Seiser C (1997) Identification of mouse histone deacetylase 1 as a growth factor-inducible gene. Mol Cell Biol 17(9):5033–5043
5. Fritsche P, Seidler B, Schuler S et al (2009) HDAC2 mediates therapeutic resistance of pancreatic cancer cells via the BH3-only protein NOXA. Gut 58(10):1399–1409
6. Trivedi CM, Luo Y, Yin Z et al (2007) Hdac2 regulates the cardiac hypertrophic response by modulating Gsk3 beta activity. Nat Med 13:324–331
7. Kook H, Lepore JJ, Gitler AD et al (2003) Cardiac hypertrophy and histone deacetylase-dependent transcriptional repression mediated by the atypical homeodomain protein hop. J Clin Invest 112:863–871
8. Kee HJ, Sohn IS, Nam KI et al (2006) Inhibition of histone deacetylation blocks cardiac hypertrophy induced by angiotensin II infusion and aortic banding. Circulation 113:51–59
9. Grabiec AM, Krausz S, de Jager W et al (2010) Histone deacetylase inhibitors suppress inflammatory activation of rheumatoid arthritis patient synovial macrophages and tissue. J Immunol 184(5):2718–2728
10. De Caro C, Di Cesare ML, Branca JJV et al (2020) Pain modulation in WAG/Rij epileptic rats (a genetic model of absence epilepsy): effects of biological and pharmacological histone deacetylase inhibitors. Front Pharmacol 3:11
11. Hajjar R, Richard CS, Santos MM (2021) The role of butyrate in surgical and oncological outcomes in colorectal cancer. Am J Physiol Gastrointest Liver Physiol 320(4):G601–G608
12. Cui SS, Yang CP, Bowen RC et al (2003) Valproic acid enhances axonal regeneration and recovery of motor function after sciatic nerve axotomy in adult rats. Brain Res 975(1–2):229–236
13. Kozubek A, Tyman JHP (1999) Resorcinolic lipids, the natural non-isoprenoid phenolic amphiphiles and their biological activity. Chem Rev 99(1):1–26
14. Kushneruk MA, Tugarova AV, Il'chukova AV et al (2013) Factors inducing transition from growth to dormancy in rhizobacteria Azospirillum brasilense. Mikrobiologiia 82(5):563–570
15. Arias E, González J, Peiró JM, Oria R, Lopez-Buesa P (2007) Browning prevention by ascorbic acid and 4-hexylresorcinol: different mechanisms of action on polyphenol oxidase in the presence and in the absence of substrates. J Food Sci 72:C464–C470
16. Chhabra RS, Huff JE, Haseman J, Hall A, Baskin G, Cowan M (1988) Inhibition of some spontaneous tumors by 4-hexylresorcinol in F344/N rats and B6C3F1 mice. Fundam Appl Toxicol 11:685–690
17. National Toxicology Program (1988) NTP toxicology and carcinogenesis studies of 4-hexylresorcinol (CAS no. 136-77-6) in F344/N rats and B6C3F1 mice (gavage studies). Natl Toxicol Program Tech Rep Ser 330:1–166

18. Kim SG, Lee SW, Park YW, Jeong JH, Choi JY (2011) 4-hexylresorcinol inhibits NF-κB phosphorylation and has a synergistic effect with cisplatin in KB cells. Oncol Rep 26:1527–1532
19. Kim SG, Kim AS, Jeong JH, Choi JY, Kweon H (2012) 4-hexylresorcinol stimulates the differentiation of SCC-9 cells through the suppression of E2F2, E2F3 and Sp3 expression and the promotion of Sp1 expression. Oncol Rep 28:677–681
20. Kim SG, Jeong JH, Park YW et al (2011) 4-hexylresorcinol inhibits transglutaminase-2 activity and has synergistic effects along with cisplatin in KB cells. Oncol Rep 25:1597–1602
21. Kweon HY, Kim SG, Choi JY (2014) Inhibition of foreign body giant cell formation by 4-hexylresorcinol through suppression of diacylglycerol kinase delta gene expression. Biomaterials 35:8576–8584
22. Ahn JH, Kim SG, Kim MK et al (2016) Topical delivery of 4-hexylresorcinol promotes wound healing via tumor necrosis factor-α suppression. Burns 42:1534–1541
23. Kim SG (2020) Immunomodulation for maxillofacial reconstructive surgery. Maxillofac Plast Reconstr Surg 42:5
24. Kim MK, Yoon CS, Kim SG, Park YW, Lee SK (2019) Effects of 4-hexylresorcinol on protein expressions in RAW 264.7 cells as determined by immunoprecipitation high performance liquid chromatography. Sci Rep 9:3379
25. Kim DW, Jo YY, Garagiola U et al (2020) Increased level of vascular endothelial growth factors by 4-hexylresorcinol is mediated by transforming growth factor-β1 and accelerates capillary regeneration in the burns in diabetic animals. Int J Mol Sci 21:3473
26. Furumai R, Komatsu Y, Nishino N, Khochbin S, Yoshida M, Horinouchi S (2001) Potent histone deacetylase inhibitors built from trichostatin a and cyclic tetrapeptide antibiotics including trapoxin. Proc Natl Acad Sci USA 98:87–92
27. Kim JY, Kweon HY, Kim DW, Choi JY, Kim SG (2021) 4-hexylresorcinol inhibits class I histone deacetylases in human umbilical cord endothelial cells. Appl Sci 11(8):3486
28. Kim MS, Kwon HJ, Lee YM et al (2001) Histone deacetylases induce angiogenesis by negative regulation of tumor suppressor genes. Nat Med 7:437–443
29. Jo YY, Kim DW, Choi JY, Kim SG (2019) 4-hexylresorcinol and silk sericin increase the expression of vascular endothelial growth factor via different pathways. Sci Rep 9:3448
30. Shukla A, Choudhury S, Chaudhary G et al (2021) Chitosan and gelatin biopolymer supplemented with mesenchymal stem cells (Velgraft®) enhanced wound healing in goats (Capra hircus): involvement of VEGF, TGF and CD31. J Tissue Viability 30:59–66
31. Zhang Y, Liu J, Zou T et al (2021) DPSCs treated by TGF-β1 regulate angiogenic sprouting of three-dimensionally co-cultured HUVECs and DPSCs through VEGF-Ang-Tie2 signaling. Stem Cell Res Ther 12:281
32. Healy SJM, Verfaillie T, Jäger R, Agostinis P, Samali A (2012) Biology of the endoplasmic reticulum. In: Agostinis P, Samali A (eds) Endoplasmic reticulum stress in health and disease. Springer, Heidelberg, pp 3–22; ISBN 978-94-007-4350-2
33. Zhou L, Liu Z, Chen S et al (2021) Transcription factor EB-mediated autophagy promotes dermal fibroblast differentiation and collagen production by regulating endoplasmic reticulum stress and autophagy-dependent secretion. Int J Mol Med 47:547–560
34. Berger E, Haller D (2011) Structure-function analysis of the tertiary bile acid TUDCA for the resolution of endoplasmic reticulum stress in intestinal epithelial cells. Biochem Biophys Res Commun 409:610–615
35. Kim JY, Kim DW, Lee SK et al (2021) Increased expression of TGF-β1 by 4-hexylresorcinol is mediated by endoplasmic reticulum and mitochondrial stress in human umbilical endothelial vein cells. Appl Sci 11(19):9128
36. Kim MK, Kim SG, Lee SK (2020) 4-hexylresorcinol-induced angiogenesis potential in human endothelial cells. Maxillofac Plast Reconstr Surg 42:23
37. Vassilopoulos A, Fritz KS, Petersen DR, Gius D (2011) The human sirtuin family: evolutionary divergences and functions. Hum Genomics 5:485–496

38. Aka JA, Kim GW, Yang XJ (2011) K-acetylation and its enzymes: overview and new developments. In: Yao TP, Seto E (eds) Histone deactylases: the biology and clinical implication. Springer, New York, NY, pp 1–12; ISBN 978-3-642-21630-5
39. Yen GC, Duh PD, Lin CW (2003) Effects of resveratrol and 4-hexylresorcinol on hydrogen peroxide-induced oxidative DNA damage in human lymphocytes. Free Radic Res 37:509–514
40. Dauer P, Gupta VK, McGinn O et al (2017) Inhibition of Sp1 prevents ER homeostasis and causes cell death by lysosomal membrane permeabilization in pancreatic cancer. Sci Rep 7:1564. https://doi.org/10.1038/s41598-017-01696-2
41. Deb DK, Chen Y, Sun J, Wang Y, Li YC (2017) ATP-citrate lyase is essential for high glucose-induced histone hyperacetylation and fibrogenic gene upregulation in mesangial cells. Am J Physiol Renal Physiol 313:F423–F429
42. Martin-Gallausiaux C, Béguet-Crespel F, Marinelli L et al (2018) Butyrate produced by gut commensal bacteria activates TGF-beta1 expression through the transcription factor SP1 in human intestinal epithelial cells. Sci Rep 8:9742
43. Amuthan G, Biswas G, Ananadatheerthavarada HK, Vijayasarathy C, Shephard HM, Avadhani NG (2002) Mitochondrial stress-induced calcium signaling, phenotypic changes and invasive behavior in human lung carcinoma A549 cells. Oncogene 21:7839–7849
44. Xu J, Kitada M, Koya D (2020) The impact of mitochondrial quality control by sirtuins on the treatment of type 2 diabetes and diabetic kidney disease. Biochim Biophys Acta Mol basis Dis 1866:165756
45. Liu J, Chen B, Hu Q, Zhang Q, Huang B, Fei P (2023) Pectin grafted with resorcinol and 4-hexylresorcinol: preparation, characterization and application in meat preservation. Int J Biol Macromol 237:124212
46. Kim YS, Kim DW, Kim SG, Lee SK (2020) 4-hexylresorcinol-induced protein expression changes in human umbilical cord vein endothelial cells as determined by immunoprecipitation high-performance liquid chromatography. PLoS One 15:e0243975
47. Harding HP, Zhang Y, Ron D (1999) Protein translation and folding are coupled by an endoplasmic-reticulum-resident kinase. Nature 397:271–274
48. Yamamoto K, Sato T, Matsui T et al (2007) Transcriptional induction of mammalian ER quality control proteins is mediated by single or combined action of ATF6alpha and XBP1. Dev Cell 13:365–376
49. Ye J, Rawson RB, Komuro R et al (2000) ER stress induces cleavage of membrane-bound ATF6 by the same proteases that process SREBPs. Mol Cell 6:1355–1364
50. Douglas PM, Summers DW, Cyr DM (2009) Molecular chaperones antagonize proteotoxicity by differentially modulating protein aggregation pathways. Prion 3:51–58
51. Lu PD, Harding HP, Ron D (2004) Translation reinitiation at alternative open reading frames regulates gene expression in an integrated stress response. J Cell Biol 167:27–33
52. PubChem. https://pubchem.ncbi.nlm.nih.gov/compound/3610. Accessed 25 Jul 2021
53. Basseri S, Austin RC (2012) Endoplasmic reticulum stress and the unfolded protein response in lipid metabolism and obesity. In: Agostinis P, Samali A (eds) Endoplasmic reticulum stress in health and disease. Springer, Heidelberg, pp 231–256; ISBN 978-94-007-4350-2
54. Lee IS, Chang JH, Kim DW, Kim SG, Kim TW (2021) The effect of 4-hexylresorcinol administration on NAD+ level and SIRT activity in Saos-2 cells. Maxillofac Plast Reconstr Surg 43:39
55. Yang Y, Sauve AA (2016) Biochemistry and enzymology of sirtuins. In: Houtkooper RH (ed) Sirtuins, proteins and cell regulation. Springer, Heidelberg, pp 1–28; ISBN 978-94-024-0961-1
56. Chu S (2012) Transcriptional regulation by post-transcriptional modification—role of phosphorylation in Sp1 transcriptional activity. Gene 508:1–8
57. Liao M, Zhang Y, Dufau ML (2008) Protein kinase calpha-induced derepression of the human luteinizing hormone receptor gene transcription through ERK mediated release of HDAC1/Sin3A repressor complex from Sp1 sites. Mol Endocrinol 22:1449–1463
58. Darlow HM, Powell EO (1957) An effect of hexylresorcinol on bacterial aerosols. Nature 180:1425–1426

59. Howitz KT, Bitterman KJ, Cohen HY et al (2003) Small molecule activators of sirtuins extend Saccharomyces cerevisiae lifespan. Nature 425:191–196
60. Civitarese AE, Carling S, Heilbronn LK et al (2007) Calorie restriction increases muscle mitochondrial biogenesis in healthy humans. PLoS Med 4:e76
61. Kincaid B, Bossy-Wetzel E (2013) Forever young: SIRT3 a shield against mitochondrial meltdown, aging, and neurodegeneration. Front Aging Neurosci 5:48
62. Zhang P, Tu B, Wang H et al (2014) Tumor suppressor p53 cooperates with SIRT6 to regulate gluconeogenesis by promoting FoxO1 nuclear exclusion. Proc Natl Acad Sci USA 111:10684–10689
63. Kim SG, Choi JY (2013) 4-hexylresorcinol exerts antitumor effects via suppression of calcium oscillation and its antitumor effects are inhibited by calcium channel blockers. Oncol Rep 29:1835–1840
64. Lee SW, Kim SG, Park YW, Kweon H, Kim JY, Rotaru H (2013) Cisplatin and 4-hexylresorcinol synergise to decrease metastasis and increase survival rate in an oral mucosal melanoma xenograft model: a preliminary study. Tumour Biol 34:1595–1603
65. Chen Y, Zhang J, Lin Y et al (2011) Tumour suppressor SIRT3 deacetylates and activates manganese superoxide dismutase to scavenge ROS. EMBO Rep 12:534–541
66. Kanfi Y, Peshti V, Gil R, Naiman S, Nahum L, Levin E (2010) SIRT6 protects against pathological damage caused by diet-induced obesity. Aging Cell 9:162–173
67. Kawahara TL, Rapicavoli NA, Wu AR, Qu K, Quake SR, Chang HY (2011) Dynamic chromatin localization of Sirt6 shapes stress- and aging-related transcriptional networks. PLoS Genet 7:e1002153
68. Song JY, Kim SG, Park NR, Choi JY (2018) Porcine bone incorporated with 4-hexylresorcinol increases new bone formation by suppression of the nuclear factor kappa B signaling pathway. J Craniofac Surg 29:1983–1990
69. Canto C, Jiang LQ, Deshmukh AS et al (2010) Interdependence of AMPK and SIRT1 for metabolic adaptation to fasting and exercise in skeletal muscle. Cell Metab 11:213–219
70. Chau MD, Gao J, Yang Q, Wu Z, Gromada J (2010) Fibroblast growth factor 21 regulates energy metabolism by activating the AMPK-SIRT1-PGC-1alpha pathway. Proc Natl Acad Sci USA 107:12553–12558
71. Rogina B, Helfand SL (2004) Sir2 mediates longevity in the fly through a pathway related to calorie restriction. Proc Natl Acad Sci USA 101:15998–16003
72. Curtin NJ, Szabo C (2013) Therapeutic applications of PARP inhibitors: anticancer therapy and beyond. Mol Asp Med 34:1217–1256
73. Jung RC (1954) Use of a hexylresorcinol tablet in the enema treatment of whipworm infection. Am J Trop Med Hyg 3:918–921
74. Martin BJ, Campbell PM, Rees TD, Buschang PH (2016) A randomized controlled trial evaluating antioxidant-essential oil gel as a treatment for gingivitis in orthodontic patients. Angle Orthod 86:407–412
75. Jang JK, Kim DW, Kim SG, Kim TW (2020) Inhibitory effects of 4-hexylresorcinol on root resorption induced by orthodontic tooth movement. Appl Sci 10:6313
76. Chang JH, Kim DW, Kim SG, Kim TW (2021) Alleviation of oxidative stress in dental pulp cells following 4-hexylresorcinol administration in a rat model. Appl Sci 11:3637
77. Sheth RD, Wesolowski CA, Jacob JC et al (1995) Effect of carbamazepine and valproate on bone mineral density. J Pediatr 127:256–262
78. Boluk A, Guzelipek M, Savli H, Temel I, Ozişik HI, Kaygusuz A (2004) The effect of valproate on bone mineral density in adult epileptic patients. Pharmacol Res 50:93–97
79. Elliott JO, Jacobson MP, Haneef Z (2007) Homocysteine and bone loss in epilepsy. Seizure 16:22–34
80. Lee IS, Kim DW, Oh JH et al (2021) Effects of 4-hexylresorcinol on craniofacial growth in rats. Int J Mol Sci 22(16):8935
81. Kim YH, Kim JM, Lee JS et al (2016) Development and validation of an analytical method for the determination of 4-hexylresorcinol in food. Food Chem 190:1086–1092

82. Amadasi A, Mozzarelli A, Meda C, Maggi A, Cozzini P (2009) Identification of xenoestrogens in food additives by an integrated in silico and in vitro approach. Chem Res Toxicol 22:52–63
83. Kang YJ, Oh JH, Seok H et al (2020) 4-hexylresorcinol exhibits different characteristics to estrogen. Appl Sci 10(5):1737
84. Noda K, Chang HP, Takahashi I, Kinoshita Z, Kawamoto T (1994) Effects of the anabolic steroid nandrolone phenylpropionate on craniofacial growth in rats. J Morphol 220:25–33
85. He S, Hartsfield JK, Guo Y, Cao Y, Wang S, Chen S (2012) Association between CYP19A1 genotype and pubertal sagittal jaw growth. Am J Orthod Dentofacial Orthop 142:662–670
86. Cho SH, Chai JH, Chang SY, Kim SA (2020) Acute valproate exposure induces sex-specific changes in steroid hormone metabolism in the cerebral cortex of juvenile mice. Neurochem Res 45:2044–2051
87. Taubøll E, Gregoraszczuk EL, Kołodziej A, Kajta M, Ropstad E (2003) Valproate inhibits the conversion of testosterone to estradiol and acts as an apoptotic agent in growing porcine ovarian follicular cells. Epilepsia 44:1014–1021
88. Gamez-Del-Estal MM, Contreras I, Prieto-Pérez R, Ruiz-Rubio M (2014) Epigenetic effect of testosterone in the behavior of C. elegans. A clue to explain androgen-dependent autistic traits? Front Cell Neurosci 8:69
89. Itzhak Y, Liddie S, Anderson KL (2013) Sodium butyrate-induced histone acetylation strengthens the expression of cocaine-associated contextual memory. Neurobiol Learn Mem 102:34–42
90. Mendonça ML, Pereira FA, Nogueira-Barbosa MH et al (2013) Increased vertebral morphometric fracture in patients with postsurgical hypoparathyroidism despite normal bone mineral density. BMC Endocr Disord 13:1
91. Hassona Y, Rajab L, Taimeh D, Scully C (2018) Sanjad-Sakati syndrome: oral health care. Med Princ Pract 27:293–296
92. Shimizu E, Selvamurugan N, Westendorf JJ, Olson EN, Partridge NC (2010) HDAC4 represses matrix metalloproteinase-13 transcription in osteoblastic cells, and parathyroid hormone controls this repression. J Biol Chem 285:9616–9626
93. Gutiérrez SJ, Gómez M, Rey JA, Ochoa M, Gutiérrez SM, Prieto JC (2010) Polymorphisms of the noggin gene and mandibular micrognathia: a first approximation. Acta Odontol Latinoam 23:13–19
94. Wójcik D, Beń-Skowronek I (2020) Craniofacial morphology in children with growth hormone deficiency and turner syndrome. Diagnostics 10(2):88
95. Wang Y, Zhu W, Chen L, Liang L (2020) Early growth hormone intervention improves glucose metabolism in adult rats born small for gestational age. Exp Clin Endocrinol Diabetes 128:125–132
96. Garcia-Villalba P, Jimenez-Lara AM, Castillo AI, Aranda A (1997) Histone acetylation influences thyroid hormone and retinoic acid-mediated gene expression. DNA Cell Biol 16:421–431

Chapter 6
The Application of 4-Hexylresorcinol for Wound Healing

Abstract This chapter discusses the potential applications of 4-hexylresorcinol (4HR) in wound healing, angiogenesis, and osteoinduction. 4HR has been shown to improve epithelialization, increase angiogenesis, and stimulate osteogenesis. Its ability to modulate the expression of transcription factors, such as Sp1, E2F, and TGF-β1, contributes to these healing processes. Additionally, 4HR has been found to have anti-inflammatory properties, further supporting its potential as a therapeutic agent. In diabetic animal models, 4HR has demonstrated positive effects on wound healing and vascular network organization. Furthermore, 4HR has shown potential in osteoinduction and dental hard tissue formation, indicating its potential use in bone grafting and dental damage repair. Overall, 4HR holds promise as a candidate for improving wound healing, angiogenesis, and bone and dental regeneration.

Keywords 4-hexylresorcinol (4HR) · Wound healing · Angiogenesis · Osteoinduction · Epithelialization · Bone grafting

Wound healing is a complicated process. Wound healing process is started from receiving injury. According to the nature of injury, the pattern of wound is different. In case of stab wound, the formation of blood clot and recruiting inflammation-associated cells are shown in early stage of wound healing. Subsequently, angiogenesis and fibrotic tissue formation are observed [1]. The regeneration of epithelial tissue is also accompanied in this stage. Finally, tissue remodeling is followed. As tissue remodeling is a relatively long-term process compared to early inflammatory phase and regeneration phase, accelerating remodelling phase may shorten overall time required for healing [2]. However, wound remodeling is very hard to differentiate to normal remodeling in heathy tissue. Unhealed wound is accompanied by chronic inflammation. Though there are many reasons for chronic inflammation, microbial infection is frequently found in chronic inflammation. Accordingly, most topical ointments for accelerating wound healing focus on reducing the infection during the inflammatory phase [3].

S.-G. Kim, *Biomedical Application of 4-Hexylresorcinol*,
https://doi.org/10.1007/978-981-97-0637-2_6

Inflammation is an inevitable process of wound healing. When injury is received, natural defense line will be broken. Consequently, the injured area receives massive attack from foreign body such as microorganism or toxic material. To neutralize this invasion, host defense system should be launched. Tissue resident macrophage is a sensor for tissue injury [4]. Tissue resident macrophage recruits blood originated immune cells. Cells reside in the injured area undergo hypoxic state due to the broken capillary chain. Hypoxic stress increases the expression level of vascular endothelial growth factor [5]. The elevated level of vascular endothelial growth factor (VEGF) in the inflammatory phase helps vasodilatation and increases vascular permeability [6]. For recruiting much more immune cells from the vascular channel, vasodilatation and increasing vascular permeability are prerequisite conditions. During inflammatory phase, destroyed intra- and extracellular components are scavenged by the macrophages. This type of cleanup is required for the transformation to the next phase. If there is any limitation in cleanup process by host cells, surgical debridement will help the wound healing [3].

The inflammation period should be short as possible as it can. The termination of the inflammation period means that there are few residual inflammation inducers. Accordingly, prolonged inflammation period implies that there is ongoing tissue destruction and delayed wound healing process [3]. Bacterial toxin or cellular lysates can increase the expression level of tumor necrosis factor-α (TNF-α) and interleukin-1β (IL1β) [7]. Though these cytokines help the recruitment of immune cells to the battlefield, they increase swelling and pain in the affected site [8]. Inflammation-induced pain and tissue destruction are main complaints of injured patients. Any reagent that can suppress inflammation may help for the patients in reducing uncomfortable symptoms. In addition, reducing excessive inflammation may help wound healing in the limited cases [9]. However, intentional suppression of inflammation may delay the wound healing via disturbing host defense mechanism.

It is important to consider wound healing acceleration beyond the suppression of inflammation. During the regenerative phase, hypoxia can lead to excessive deposition of fibrotic tissue and keloid formation [10]. Thus, it is necessary to regulate the expression of transforming growth factor-β1 (TGF-β1) during the regeneration and remodeling phase, as well as to activate matrix degrading enzymes such as matrix metalloproteinase (MMP) [11]. Additionally, cellular differentiation and angiogenesis should be activated without concern for carcinogenesis.

4-Hexylresorcinol (4HR) is a chemical chaperone and has beneficial properties in the wound healing [12]. The administration of 4HR can improve cellular differentiation and angiogenesis [13]. In case of bone defect, many proteins that are important for osteogenesis can have increased expression level by 4HR administration [14].

6.1 4HR Increases Cellular Differentiation

The features of differentiated cell compared to proliferating cell are reduced cellular metabolism and mitosis. Though microbial dormancy is the different state of terminally differentiated eukaryotic cell, the similarities are no mitosis and low metabolism. The key feature of chemical chaperone is inducing dormancy in the microorganism [15]. As 4HR is a chemical chaperone and has species nonspecific effect, the administration of 4HR on epithelial cell may induce the phase transformation [12]. However, the differentiation of eukaryotic cell is not that simple. Even the definition of the differentiation is unclear. In case of human, single cell is a starting point, and the cell in the epithelial basal layer has definitive destination and relatively differentiated compared to fertilized oocyte. But it is hard to say that this cell is terminally differentiated because this cell can do cellular division and provide more differentiated cell continuously. Accordingly, there are several stations before destination of terminal differentiation [16].

Several transcription factors have been shown to be involved in cellular differentiation, with p53 and specificity protein 1 (Sp1) being two of the most relevant. The administration of 4HR has been reported to generally increase the activity of both p53 and Sp1 [17, 18], and both transcription factors have been associated with osteogenesis and epithelialization [19]. Additionally, both transcription factors are often found to be overexpressed in tumours, although this is not always directly linked to an overactivation of their function in the context of wound healing. For example, p53 is usually associated with cellular apoptosis in healthy cells under stress [20], but in tumors, p53 is frequently mutated and overexpressed, leading to a lack of apoptosis and instead, the maintenance of the tumor microenvironment [21]. The complexity of the intracellular signaling pathways involved in cellular processes means that to achieve a desirable outcome, it is important to consider the co-activation or suppression of multiple signaling molecules in tandem.

Sp1 is a transcription factor that is expressed in a variety of cell types, including during spermatogenesis, where it is involved in germ cell differentiation [22]. In addition, Sp1 is highly expressed in malignant tumors, and its expression has been associated with poor prognosis [23–25], making it a potential target for cancer treatment. However, these trials have been largely unsuccessful, likely because Sp1 is involved in the activation of both oncogenes and tumor suppressor genes [26]. Thus, it is important to consider the simultaneous control of proteins that are co-activated with Sp1 in order to obtain a desirable outcome (Fig. 6.1).

As shown in Chap. 3, elevated expression of Sp1 with suppressing early2 factor (E2F) is important in the epithelial differentiation. The expression level of E2F family is generally upregulated in many types of cancer [27–29]. In case of keratinocyte, the inhibition of E2F family is prerequisite for cellular differentiation [30]. Interestingly, the administration of 4HR inhibits E2F2 and E2F3 in oral carcinoma cell [17]. The inhibition of E2F2 and E2F3 expression by 4HR administration increases the expression level of epithelial differentiation markers such as keratin 10 and involucrin [17]. Even the expression level of Sp1 is generally elevated in the cancer, the target therapy against Sp1 has not been successful in clinical trials of the cancer treatment [26]. However, it may be helpful in wound healing because certain level of cellular proliferation is required for wound healing. When it is combined with suppression of E2F family, wound healing will be more desirable compared to keloid formation. As shown above, 4HR suppresses the expression level of E2F family [17]. The administration of 4HR can increase the expression level of Sp1 and its transcription activity [31]. Topical application of 4HR ointment shows accelerated epithelialization compared to untreated or negative control group [32].

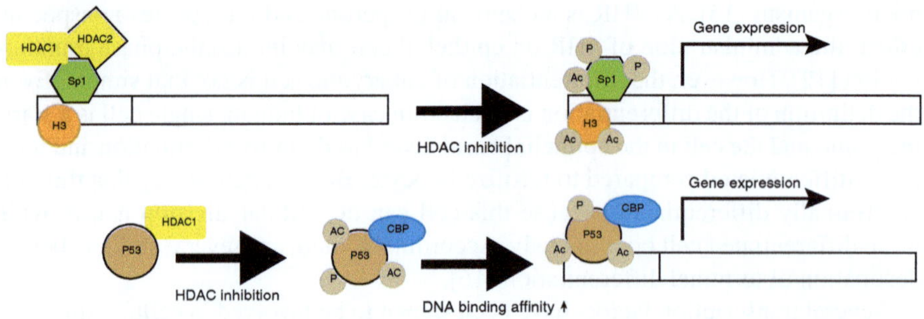

Fig. 6.1 Schematic model showing the activation of gene transcription by the administration of HDAC inhibitor. Sp1 is an inactive state when it is associated with HDAC1 and HDAC2. The administration of HDAC inhibitor will increase the acetylation level of Sp1 and H3. On contrary, HDAC1 and HDAC2 are dissociated with Sp1. Other cofactors can be recruited and stabilize the acetylated and phosphorylated Sp1. P53 can be activated with similar pattern. P52 is an inactive state when it is associated with HDAC1. P53 can be acetylated by the administration of HDAC inhibitor. CBP is cofactor for the stabilization and binding to the target DNA. Consequently, the target gene transcription can be started

In the skin injury, the loss of epithelium is observed. For the epithelial wound, keratinocyte migration to the injured area is an important step during healing process. If keratinocyte migration is inhibited, wound healing will be impaired [33]. TGF-β1 is a key cytokine involved in all phase of wound healing [34]. In the early phase of injury, TGF-β1 is released from blood clot and plays a role as chemoattractant for hiring leukocytes. The impaired wound healing is frequent complication of diabetes and it is associated with low expression level of TGF-β1 [35]. The application of TGF-β1 can accelerates keratinocyte migration and helps re-epithelialization in skin wound of animal model [36]. However, direct application of TGF-β1 on human has not been successful [37]. As TGF-β1 is a strong chemotactic cytokine, TGF-β1 is involved in the initiation and maintenance of inflammation [38]. Accordingly, the elevated expression level of TGF-β1 should accompany the inhibition of excessive inflammation to promote wound healing. The administration of 4HR increases expression level of TGF-β1 in many cell types [31, 39]. As 4HR inhibits nuclear factor κ-light-chain-enhancer of activated B cells (NF-κB) pathway [40] and the expression of tumor necrosis factor-α (TNF-α) [41], 4HR has anti-inflammatory property. Combined action of TGF-β1 activation and anti-inflammation, the application of 4HR ointment improves epithelial burn wound healing in the diabetic animal model [32].

6.2 4HR Increases Angiogenesis

Many eukaryote cells have mitochondria in their cytoplasm. Oxygen is an essential element for the mitochondrial respiration. Blood vessel is the main route for the delivery of oxygen to cells. Thus, oxygen deficiency is the main deriving force for angiogenesis. Without angiogenesis, wound healing should be impaired [1]. VEGF is an important cytokine for angiogenesis [4]. Hypoxia is an oxygen-deficient state. The expression level of hypoxia-inducible factor (HIF) is elevated in hypoxic state [42]. HIF is a strong inducer for VEGF [43].

Elevated expression level of VEGF is observed in both early and late stages of injury [44]. VEGF increases vascular permeability and induces vasodilatation in early stage of injury [6]. Compared to capillary regeneration, vasodilatation is a smart strategy for speedy supply of oxygen and nutrient in injured area. However, this reaction induces tissue destruction and swelling due to osmotic pressure. In phase transformation from inflammation to regeneration, tissue-resident macrophage plays an important role [4]. M2 type of macrophages are predominant in the regeneration phase [45]. M2-type macrophages express TGF-β1 and MMPs for cellular proliferation and differentiation [46].

In our previous study, the application of 4HR on RAW264.7 cell and HUVEC increases VEGF via HIF-independent pathway [13, 47]. Increased angiogenesis by 4HR administration is mainly mediated by TGF-β1 [42]. The application of TGF-β1 siRNA decreases 4HR-induced VEGF expression in HUVEC [42]. Topical delivery of TGF-β1 gene helps early wound closure and angiogenesis in diabetic animal model [48]. The application of TGF-β1 on stem cell induces cellular differentiation [49].

Sp1 is important in endoplasmic reticulum (ER) homeostasis [50]. As shown above, TGF-β1 is broadly expressed through whole wound healing process. The activation of Sp1 by phosphorylation increases the expression level of TGF-β1 [51]. The phosphorylated Sp1 and Sp1 transcription activity is increased by 4HR administration in HUVEC [32]. When Sp1 inhibitor (mithramycin) is treated before 4HR administration, 4HR-induced TGF-β1 expression is decreased [32].

Histone deacetylase (HDAC) is an enzyme removing acetyl group from the proteins such as histone [52]. The inhibition of HDAC increases the acetylation level of the histone and the expression level of target genes via relaxation of the chromatin. Interestingly, few genes (1–7%) are influenced their expression by the administration of histone deacetylase inhibitor (HDACi) [53, 54]. The administration of HDACi can increase the expression level of Sp1 [55]. Trichostatin A and suberoylanilide hydroxamic acid are widely studied HDACi, and the administration of these chemicals can elevate the expression level of TGF-β1 expression [56]. As shown above, 4HR can increase the expression level of Sp1 via HDACi activity [32]. The acetylation level of histone 3 (H3) is important for the transcription of TGF-β1 [57]. The administration of 4HR increases the acetylation level of H3 (Fig. 6.1).

As 4HR is a chemical chaperone, its administration should change the protein conformation as more stabilized form [12]. Any chemical reagent that can induce protein folding change can induce ER stress. Accordingly, 4HR can induce ER stress as dose-dependent manner [31]. The affinity to 4HR can be different to protein structure. Using 4HR-incorporated bead, high-performance liquid chromatography (HPLC) can filter target proteins of 4HR in RAW264.7 cell [47]. As results, many proteins are found to bind to 4HR. They are associated with the inhibition of proliferation [47]. When similar study is done for endothelial cell, the proteins associated with cellular differentiation and cellular protection show increased expression level such as TGF-β1, suppressor of mothers against decapentaplegic2/3 (SMAD2/3), and rat sarcoma (RAS) signaling protein [58]. These proteins are closely associated with 4HR-induced angiogenesis.

When misfolded protein is found in the cell, glucose-regulated protein 78 (GRP78) detects misfolded protein and tags on it [59]. GRP78-tagged protein is transported to ER and activates protein kinase R (PKR)-like endoplasmic reticulum kinase (PERK) and activates transcription factor 4 (ATF4) [60]. As 4HR decreases oxidative respiration of mitochondria, ATP synthesis in the mitochondria is slightly decreased by 4HR administration [12]. As glycolysis and lactate dehydrogenase activity are increased by 4HR administration, the level of nicotinamide adenine dinucleotide (NAD+) is upregulated [61]. Sirtuin (SIRT) is important in cellular survival, and the expression level of SIRT is elevated by reduced ATP synthesis with increasing NAD+ level [62]. The administration of 4HR can increase the expression level of SIRT and its activity [31].

4HR is a dormancy inducer for active proliferating microorganism [63]. Many live organisms try to proliferate in the favorable environment, any chemical-inhibiting proliferation should induce enough stress to stop it. Accordingly, the administered 4HR on the proliferating microorganism can behave as antiseptic [64]. Few microorganisms can survive from 4HR administration and undergo a state of dormancy. The microorganism in the dormancy can resist much harsh environmental stress [63, 65]. Considering species non-specific effect of 4HR, the administration of 4HR will not result in cellular proliferation. Thus, TGF-β1 induced by 4HR administration cannot behave as activator of cellular proliferation shown in the inflammation. Co-activated signaling pathway with TGF-β1 by 4HR administration will guide the cell to the differentiated state. Tauroursodeoxycholate (TUDCA) has been considered as suppressing agent against ER stress [66]. TUDCA has both hydrophilic and hydrophobic domains like 4HR and is claimed as a chemical chaperone [66]. Chemical chaperone can be defined as "a small molecule can bind to the proteins for stabilizing their structure from the environmental stress." If TUDCA is chemical chaperone, it should bind to protein and change its conformation. In this case, the generation of ER stress is inevitable consequence, and the intensity of ER stress only matters. After binding chemical chaperone to its target proteins, target proteins can resist high harsh environmental stress such as radiation [67]. In this case, chemical chaperone can be mentioned as stress reliever. Thus, any claim that chemical chaperone can reduce ER stress should be interpreted carefully.

With the administration of 4HR in the diabetic animal model, more organized vascular network is observed compared to the administration of sericin (Fig. 6.2). Both 4HR and sericin can increase the expression level of VEGF [42]. Both VEGF and TGF-β1 are expressed highly in both inflammatory phase and proliferating/remodeling phase [68]. Inducing differentiation and mature vessel formation by 4HR administration can be used for the development of vascular patch. It will be discussed later.

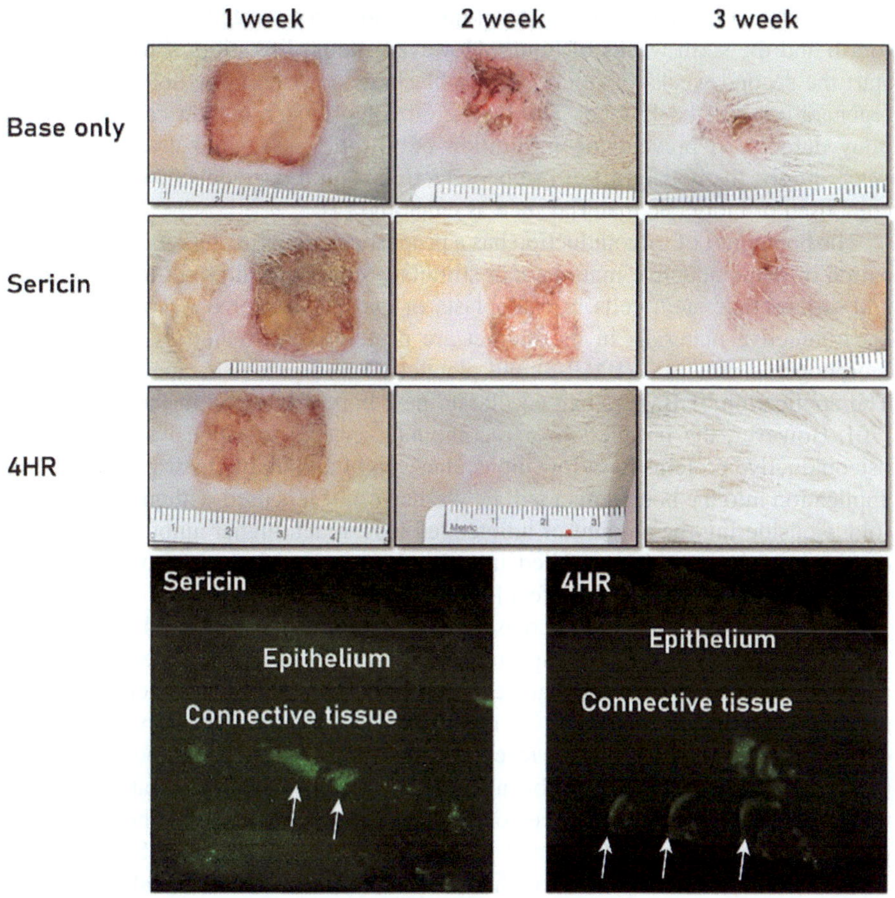

Fig. 6.2 Burn wound healing in the streptozotocin-induced diabetic animal model. Compared to base (lanolin oil) and sericin application, 4HR ointment shows speedy epithelialization. Using fluorescent dye, capillary regeneration is checked. Vasodilatation is evident in sericin group (arrows). Sprouting vessels from the deep area of connective tissue (arrows) are observed in 4HR group (Edited from author's previous publication [32])

6.3 Osteoinduction by 4HR

Bone defect is frequently observed in the head and facial injury. In case of critical sized defect, whole defect volume cannot be regenerated by new bone formation. Residual bony defect volume is usually replaced by fibrotic tissue. This incomplete regeneration is a problem in subsequent functional rehabilitation. In this case, bone graft is required [14].

According to the nature of bone graft, the property of graft can be classified as osteoconduction and osteoinduction [69]. The material having osteoconduction property is used for the volume replacement concept. The osteoblasts migrate into the bony defect from the third weeks of injury and start the calcification between the fourth and the sixth weeks of injury. However, the proliferation of fibroblasts can start the second weeks of injury. If fibroblasts occupy the bony defect, new bone regeneration will be limited. The bone graft of osteoconduction can occupy the bony defect and prevent the infiltration of fibrotic tissue into the bony defect. Accordingly, the bone graft of osteoconduction should degrade slowly and mainly composed of inorganic material such as calcium [14].

The bone graft of osteoinduction has a property as signaling molecule. The application of osteoinductive material can stimulate stem cells adjacent to bony defect and differentiate stem cells to osteoblasts or endothelial cells. Accordingly, most osteoinductive materials in the market are protein-based materials such as bone morphogenic protein-2 (BMP-2) and platelet-derived growth factor (PDGF) [14]. The application of BMP-2 can accelerate new bone formation in the bony defect [70]. However, the production of recombinant protein is expensive. In addition, osteoinductive proteins have low molecular weight and highly hydrophilic [71]. Its application into the bony defect will be washed out if it is used without proper scaffold. Considering the amount of unintended loss, much higher amount of osteoinductive protein should be applied into the defect. Overdosage of osteoinductive protein may induce off-target effect [70].

As shown above, 4HR can increase the expression level of Sp1 and p53 [18, 31]. Both transcription factors are important in odontogenesis and osteogenesis [19]. In addition, Sp1 and p53 can regulate key transcription factors for osteogenesis such as runt-related transcription factor 2 (runx2) and osterix [19]. The administration of 4HR can increase the expression level of runx2 and osterix in dental pulp cells [39]. 4HR-incorpated bone graft has been shown successful bone regeneration [40]. As there are many similarities between osteogenesis and odontogenesis, the application of 4HR may increase the formation of dental hard tissue (Fig. 6.3). Subcutaneous injection of 4HR accelerates dental hard tissue formation in the animal model [39]. In case of dental damage model, the healing of dental pulp is improved by 4HR ointment application [72].

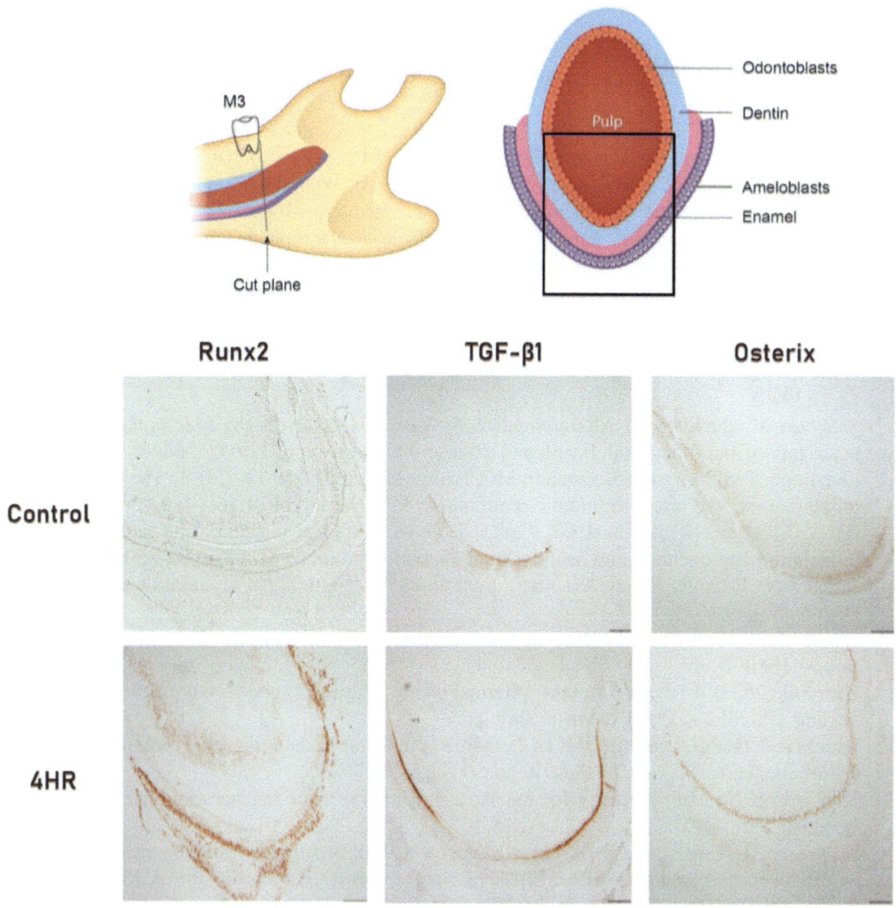

Fig. 6.3 4HR is injected to the submental area of the rats. Consequently, the expression levels of runx2, TGF-β1, and osterix are increased in the incisor root apex area compared to the untreated control (Edited from author's previous publication [39])

6.4 Closing Remark

In this chapter, the administration of 4HR can accelerate wound healing in both epithelial and bone injury. The wound healing promotion by 4HR is mainly mediated by Sp1 and p53. Additionally, the inhibition of HDAC and anti-inflammatory action will be helpful for rapid wound healing. Though TGF-β1 plays a central role in 4HR-mediated wound healing, off-target effect of TGF-β1 is controlled by co-activated signaling pathway. Using beneficial property of 4HR on wound healing, 4HR-incorprated materials can be used for tissue engineering. Its application on tissue engineering will be discussed in subsequent chapter.

References

1. Cohen IK, McCoy BJ, Diegelmann RF (1979) An update on wound healing. Ann Plast Surg 3(3):264–272
2. Nour S, Baheiraei N, Imani R et al (2019) A review of accelerated wound healing approaches: biomaterial- assisted tissue remodeling. J Mater Sci Mater Med 30(10):120
3. Powers JG, Higham C, Broussard K, Phillips TJ (2016) Wound healing and treating wounds: chronic wound care and management. J Am Acad Dermatol 74(4):607–625
4. Willenborg S, Injarabian L, Eming SA (2022) Role of macrophages in wound healing. Cold Spring Harb Perspect Biol 14(12):a041216
5. Gilkes DM, Semenza GL (2013) Role of hypoxia-inducible factors in breast cancer metastasis. Future Oncol 9(11):1623–1636
6. Vuorio T, Jauhiainen S, Ylä-Herttuala S (2012) Pro- and anti-angiogenic therapy and atherosclerosis with special emphasis on vascular endothelial growth factors. Expert Opin Biol Ther 12(1):79–92
7. Shapouri-Moghaddam A, Mohammadian S, Vazini H et al (2018) Macrophage plasticity, polarization, and function in health and disease. J Cell Physiol 233:6425–6440
8. Lenzlinger PM, Morganti-Kossmann MC, Laurer HL, McIntosh TK (2001) The duality of the inflammatory response to traumatic brain injury. Mol Neurobiol 24:169–181
9. Rai V, Moellmer R, Agrawal DK (2023) Role of fibroblast plasticity and heterogeneity in modulating angiogenesis and healing in the diabetic foot ulcer. Mol Biol Rep 50:1913–1929
10. Jumper N, Paus R, Bayat A (2015) Functional histopathology of keloid disease. Histol Histopathol 30:1033–1057
11. Chang M, Nguyen TT (2021) Strategy for treatment of infected diabetic foot ulcers. Acc Chem Res 54:1080–1093
12. Kim SG (2022) 4-hexylresorcinol: pharmacologic chaperone and its application for wound healing. Maxillofac Plast Reconstr Surg 44:5
13. Kim MK, Kim SG, Lee SK (2020) 4-hexylresorcinol-induced angiogenesis potential in human endothelial cells. Maxillofac Plast Reconstr Surg 42:23
14. Kim SG (2022) Multiple ways for the same destination: bone regeneration. Maxillofac Plast Reconstr Surg 44:9
15. Kolpakov AI, Il'inskaia ON, Bespalov MM et al (2000) Stabilization of enzymes by anabiosis autoinducers as a possible mechanism of resistance of resting microbial forms. Mikrobiologiia 69:224–230
16. DiMario JX (2002) Activation and repression of growth factor receptor gene transcription (review). Int J Mol Med 10:65–71
17. Kim SG, Kim AS, Jeong JH, Choi JY, Kweon H (2012) 4-hexylresorcinol stimulates the differentiation of SCC-9 cells through the suppression of E2F2, E2F3 and Sp3 expression and the promotion of Sp1 expression. Oncol Rep 28:677–681
18. Kang YJ, Yang WG, Chae WS, Kim DW, Kim SG, Rotaru H (2022) Administration of 4-hexylresorcinol increases p53-mediated transcriptional activity in oral cancer cells with the p53 mutation. Oncol Rep 48:160
19. Viale-Bouroncle S, Felthaus O, Schmalz G, Reichert TE, Morsczeck C (2013) Transcription factors for dental stem cell differentiation. Int J Oral Maxillofac Implants 28:e478–e486
20. Wang P, Wang HY, Gao XJ, Zhu HX, Zhang XP, Liu F, Wang W (2023) Encoding and decoding of p53 dynamics in cellular response to stresses. Cell 12:490
21. Asl ER, Rostamzadeh D, Duijf PHG et al (2023) Mutant P53 in the formation and progression of the tumor microenvironment: friend or foe. Life Sci 315:121361
22. Thomas K, Wu J, Sung DY et al (2007) SP1 transcription factors in male germ cell development and differentiation. Mol Cell Endocrinol 270:1–7
23. Aka JA, Kim GW, Yang XJ (2002) Histone deacetylases: the biology and clinical. BMC Cancer 2:35

24. Wang L, Wei D, Huang S et al (2003) Transcription factor Sp1 expression is a significant predictor of survival in human gastric cancer. Clin Cancer Res 9:6371–6380
25. Jiang NY, Woda BA, Banner BF, Whalen GF, Dresser KA, Lu D (2008) Sp1, a new biomarker that identifies a subset of aggressive pancreatic ductal adenocarcinoma. Cancer Epidemiol Biomarkers Prev 17:1648–1652
26. Beishline K, Azizkhan-Clifford J (2015) Sp1 and the 'hallmarks of cancer'. FEBS J 282:224–258
27. Liu ZL, Bi XW, Liu PP et al (2018) Expressions and prognostic values of the E2F transcription factors in human breast carcinoma. Cancer Manag Res 10:3521–3532
28. Ye WY, Lu HP, Li JD et al (2021) Clinical implication of E2F transcription factor 1 in hepatocellular carcinoma tissues. Cancer Biother Radiopharm 38:684. https://doi.org/10.1089/cbr.2020.4342
29. Zhang Y, Lyu L, Wang W, Zhang L (2022) High expression of E2F transcription factors 7: an independent predictor of poor prognosis in patients with lung adenocarcinoma. Medicine (Baltimore) 101:e29253
30. Endo-Munoz L, Dahler A, Teakle N et al (2009) E2F7 can regulate proliferation, differentiation, and apoptotic responses in human keratinocytes: implications for cutaneous squamous cell carcinoma formation. Cancer Res 69:1800–1808
31. Kim JY, Kim DW, Lee SK et al (2021) Increased expression of TGF-β1 by 4-hexylresorcinol is mediated by endoplasmic reticulum and mitochondrial stress in human umbilical endothelial vein cells. Appl Sci 11(19):9128
32. Kim DW, Jo YY, Garagiola U et al (2020) Increased level of vascular endothelial growth factors by 4-hexylresorcinol is mediated by transforming growth factor-β1 and accelerates capillary regeneration in the burns in diabetic animals. Int J Mol Sci 21(10):3473
33. Sivamani RK, Garcia MS, Isseroff RR (2007) Wound re-epithelialization: modulating keratinocyte migration in wound healing. Front Biosci 12:2849–2868
34. O'Kane S, Ferguson MW (1997) Transforming growth factor beta s and wound healing. Int J Biochem Cell Biol 29:63–78
35. Jude EB, Blakytny R, Bulmer J, Boulton AJ, Ferguson MW (2002) Transforming growth factor-beta 1, 2, 3 and receptor type I and II in diabetic foot ulcers. Diabet Med 19:440–447
36. Wang XJ, Han G, Owens P, Siddiqui Y, Li AG (2006) Role of TGF beta-mediated inflammation in cutaneous wound healing. J Investig Dermatol Symp Proc 11(1):112–117
37. Bennett SP, Griffiths GD, Schor AM, Leese GP, Schor SL (2003) Growth factors in the treatment of diabetic foot ulcers. Br J Surg 90:133–146
38. Wahl SM (1994) Transforming growth factor beta: the good, the bad, and the ugly. J Exp Med 180:1587–1590
39. Kim JH, Kim DW, Kim SG, Kim TW (2020) 4-hexylresorcinol administration increases dental hard tissue formation and incisor eruption rate in rats. Appl Sci 10(16):5511
40. Song JY, Kim SG, Park NR, Choi JY (2018) Porcine bone incorporated with 4-hexylresorcinol increases new bone formation by suppression of the nuclear factor kappa B signaling pathway. J Craniofac Surg 29(7):1983–1990
41. Ahn J, Kim SG, Kim MK et al (2016) Topical delivery of 4-hexylresorcinol promotes wound healing via tumor necrosis factor-α suppression. Burns 42(7):1534–1541
42. Steiner CA, Cartwright IM, Taylor CT, Colgan SP (2022) Hypoxia-inducible factor as a bridge between healthy barrier function, wound healing, and fibrosis. Am J Physiol Cell Physiol 323(3):C866–C878
43. Long HQ, Li GS, Cheng X, Xu JH, Li FB (2015) Role of hypoxia-induced VEGF in blood-spinal cord barrier disruption in chronic spinal cord injury. Chin J Traumatol 18(5):293–295
44. Miatmoko A, Hariawan BS, Cahyani DM et al (2023) Prospective use of amniotic mesenchymal stem cell metabolite products for tissue regeneration. J Biol Eng 17(1):11
45. Xiao W, Yang Y, Chu C et al (2023) Macrophage response mediated by extracellular matrix: recent progress. Biomed Mater 18(1):012003

46. Kim SG (2020) Immunomodulation for maxillofacial reconstructive surgery. Maxillofac Plast Reconstr Surg 42:5
47. Kim MK, Yoon CS, Kim SG, Park YW, Lee SS, Lee SK (2019) Effects of 4-hexylresorcinol on protein expressions in RAW 264.7 cells as determined by immunoprecipitation high performance liquid chromatography. Sci Rep 9:3379
48. Lee PY, Chesnoy S, Huang L (2004) Electroporatic delivery of TGF-beta1 gene works synergistically with electric therapy to enhance diabetic wound healing in db/db mice. J Invest Dermatol 123:791–798
49. Zhang X, Wang G, Wang W et al (2023) Bone marrow mesenchymal stem cells paracrine TGF-β1 to mediate the biological activity of osteoblasts in bone repair. Cytokine 164:156139
50. Dauer P, Gupta VK, McGinn O et al (2017) Inhibition of Sp1 prevents ER homeostasis and causes cell death by lysosomal membrane permeabilization in pancreatic cancer. Sci Rep 7:1564
51. Shu B, Zhang RZ, Zhou YX, He C, Yang X (2022) METTL3-mediated macrophage exosomal NEAT1 contributes to hepatic fibrosis progression through Sp1/TGF-β1/Smad signaling pathway. Cell Death Discov 8:266
52. Kim JY, Kweon HY, Kim DW, Choi JY, Kim SG (2021) 4-hexylresorcinol inhibits class I histone deacetylases in human umbilical cord endothelial cells. Appl Sci 11:3486
53. Zhu WG, Lakshmanan RR, Beal MD, Otterson GA (2001) DNA methyltransferase inhibition enhances apoptosis induced by histone deacetylase inhibitors. Cancer Res 61:1327–1333
54. Marks PA, Richon VM, Rifkind RA (2000) Histone deacetylase inhibitors: inducers of differentiation or apoptosis of transformed cells. J Natl Cancer Inst 92:1210–1216
55. Hepp MI, Escobar D, Farkas C et al (2018) A Trichostatin a (TSA)/Sp1-mediated mechanism for the regulation of SALL2 tumor suppressor in Jurkat T cells. Biochim Biophys Acta Gene Regul Mech 1861(7):623–636
56. Koppaka V, Lakshman N, Petroll WM (2015) Effect of HDAC inhibitors on corneal keratocyte mechanical phenotypes in 3-D collagen matrices. Mol Vis 21:502–514
57. Park HJ, Jeong OY, Chun SH et al (2021) Butyrate improves skin/lung fibrosis and intestinal dysbiosis in bleomycin-induced mouse models. Int J Mol Sci 22:2765
58. Kim YS, Kim DW, Kim SG, Lee SK (2020) 4-hexylresorcinol-induced protein expression changes in human umbilical cord vein endothelial cells as determined by immunoprecipitation high-performance liquid chromatography. PLoS One 15(12):e0243975
59. Hernandez I, Cohen M (2022) Linking cell-surface GRP78 to cancer: from basic research to clinical value of GRP78 antibodies. Cancer Lett 524:1–14
60. Garcia-Carbonero N, Li W, Cabeza-Morales M, Martinez-Useros J, Garcia-Foncillas J (2018) New hope for pancreatic ductal adenocarcinoma treatment targeting endoplasmic reticulum stress response: a systematic review. Int J Mol Sci 19(9):2468
61. Lee IS, Chang JH, Kim DW, Kim SG, Kim TW (2021) The effect of 4-hexylresorinol administration on NAD+ level and SIRT activity in Saos-2 cells. Maxillofac Plast Reconstr Surg 43:39
62. Lin S, Xing H, Zang T, Ruan X, Wo L, He M (2018) Sirtuins in mitochondrial stress: indispensable helpers behind the scenes. Ageing Res Rev 44:22–32
63. Kushneruk MA, Tugarova AV, Il'chukova AV et al (2013) Factors inducing transition from growth to dormancy in rhizobacteria Azospirillum brasilense. Microbiology 82:572–578
64. Musto JD, Sane JN, Warner VD (1979) Quantitative determination of hexylresorcinol in commercial antiseptic solution by high-pressure liquid chromatography. J Pharm Sci 68(2):240–241
65. Tereshkin EV, Loiko NG, Tereshkina KB, Kovalenko VV, Krupyanskii YF (2022) Possible mechanisms of 4-hexylresorcinol influence on DNA and DNA–Dps nanocrystals affecting stress sustainability of Escherichia coli. Russ J Phys Chem B 16(4):726–737
66. Kusaczuk M (2019) Tauroursodeoxycholate-bile acid with chaperoning activity: molecular and cellular effects and therapeutic perspectives. Cell 8(12):1471
67. Davydova O, Deryabin D, El'-Registan G (2006) Influence of chemical analogues of microbial autoregulators on the sensitivity of DNA to UV radiation. Microbiology 75(5):654–661

68. Pan X, You C, Wu P, Wang X, Han C (2023) The optimization of PLGA knitted mesh reinforced-collagen/chitosan scaffold for the healing of full-thickness skin defects. J Biomed Mater Res B Appl Biomater 111(4):763–774
69. Li M, Yin S, Lin M et al (2022) Current status and prospects of metal-organic frameworks for bone therapy and bone repair. J Mater Chem B 10(27):5105–5128
70. Czech T, Oyewumi MO (2021) Overcoming barriers confronting application of protein therapeutics in bone fracture healing. Drug Deliv Transl Res 11(3):842–865
71. Teng F, Yu D, Wei L, Su N, Liu Y (2019) Preclinical application of recombinant human bone morphogenetic protein 2 on bone substitutes for vertical bone augmentation: a systematic review and meta-analysis. J Prosthet Dent 122(4):355–363
72. Chang JH, Kim DW, Kim SG, Kim TW (2021) Alleviation of oxidative stress in dental pulp cells following 4-hexylresorcinol administration in a rat model. Appl Sci 11:3637–3649

Chapter 7
The Application of 4-Hexylresorcinol in Tissue Engineering

Abstract This chapter explores the potential applications of 4-hexylresorcinol (4HR) in tissue engineering, focusing on its use in silk fibroin membrane (SFM), bone graft materials, vessel regeneration, and inhibition of foreign body reactions. The incorporation of 4HR into SFM demonstrated improved bone regeneration and an acceleration of partial degradation of the SFM. However, further research is required to determine if complete resorption can be achieved. Additionally, the chapter discusses the development of 4HR-incorporated bone graft materials, including the combination of 4HR with hydroxyapatite, porcine bone, bovine bone, and sericin. These materials show promising results in enhancing bone formation and vessel regeneration while inhibiting foreign body reactions. Despite these promising findings, more research and human clinical trials are necessary to confirm their efficacy and safety. Overall, this chapter highlights the potential of 4HR-incorporated materials in tissue engineering and provides a foundation for future investigations in this area.

Keywords 4-hexylresorcinol (4HR) · Tissue engineering · Silk fibroin · Bone graft material · Foreign body reaction · Degradation

The process of repairing damaged tissue typically involves the use of graft materials. Although autogenous grafts are often considered the gold standard, the limited availability and donor site morbidity associated with autogenous grafts can be significant limitations. In contrast, alloplastic grafts can be produced as needed for the recipient and do not have the same donor site morbidity concerns. However, since alloplastic materials are foreign to the recipient, immune reactions after grafting are an unavoidable occurrence. As such, the development of alloplastic materials must prioritize minimizing immune-related issues and promoting the regeneration of tissue as required.

The host's response to a graft can vary depending on the anatomical location, as well as the composition of the graft itself, which can impact immune reactions [1]. As a result, graft materials must be tailored to meet the specific requirements of the anatomical site. To achieve desirable effects after grafting, bioactive molecules can

S.-G. Kim, *Biomedical Application of 4-Hexylresorcinol*,
https://doi.org/10.1007/978-981-97-0637-2_7

be added to the graft. Since grafting is a type of volume replacement therapy, the graft material should have sufficient volume to fill the defect [2]. Therefore, a combination of scaffold and bioactive molecules can be utilized as a graft material.

When designing an optimal biomaterial for wound healing, several conditions must be considered. Firstly, the speed at which the bioactive molecule is released from the scaffold is crucial [3]. Secondly, the rate at which the scaffold biodegrades is also an important factor to be considered [4]. Moreover, the release pattern of the bioactive molecule is dependent on the partner cells such as blood-originated cells, epithelial cells, and connective tissue-originated cells [5]. Similarly, the degradation velocity of the scaffold is also influenced by the healing rate of the host tissue [6].

The integration of 4-hexylresorcinol (4HR) into biomaterials is still under development, and its potential benefits are being explored. As 4HR possesses anti-inflammatory and antiseptic properties, its incorporation into grafts could potentially prevent inflammation and infections [7, 8]. To this end, 4HR has been integrated into silk protein-based biomaterials, which typically degrade slowly and can induce inflammation at the grafting site [9, 10]. Throughout the course of the project, various advantageous properties of incorporating 4HR into biomaterials have been uncovered.

7.1 Inhibition of Foreign Body Reaction of Graft

Foreign body giant cells (FBGCs) are multinucleated cells that are formed in response to the presence of foreign materials, such as synthetic polymers or biomaterials, in the body [11]. These cells are typically observed at the interface between the biomaterial and the host tissue.

The formation of FBGCs is a complex process that involves several steps, including initial recognition of the foreign material by phagocytic cells, phagocytosis of the material, and subsequent fusion of the phagocytic cells to form multinucleated FBGCs [12, 13]. The exact mechanisms that lead to FBGC formation are not fully understood, but there are several potential factors that have been proposed to contribute to this process. Several studies have shown that exposure to foreign materials can increase the production of reactive oxygen species (ROS) in macrophages, and that high levels of ROS can lead to the formation of FBGCs [14]. ROS are highly reactive molecules that are produced by cells as a natural part of their metabolism, but they can also be produced in response to stress or inflammation [15]. ROS can modulate macrophage polarization and fusion by regulating cytokine production and expression of co-stimulatory molecules [12]. ROS-responsive biomaterials can release drugs or other agents to modulate the tissue microenvironment and reduce inflammation and FBGC formation [16]. Different types of ROS-based biomaterials that can promote tissue regeneration and healing by influencing cellular behaviors such as proliferation, differentiation, migration, and apoptosis [17].

The exact mechanism by which ROS contribute to FBGC formation is not fully understood, but it has been suggested that ROS may trigger signaling pathways that promote cell fusion. ROS can also cause oxidative damage to proteins and lipids, which may alter the membrane properties of macrophages and facilitate fusion [18]. However, there has been no direct evidence that ROS facilitate fusion specifically in macrophages. Some studies suggest that antioxidants can reduce ROS levels and prevent oxidative damage to cells and tissues [19]. Incorporating antioxidants into a graft material may have the potential to reduce the formation of FBGCs by reducing the production of ROS in macrophages (Fig. 7.1). Antioxidants are molecules that can neutralize ROS and prevent oxidative damage to cells [20] and have been shown to be effective in reducing the formation of FBGCs in some studies. For example, one study found that incorporating an antioxidant, such as vitamin E, into a polymer scaffold reduced the production of ROS in macrophages and led to a reduction in FBGC formation [12]. Another study showed that coating a biomaterial with an antioxidant, such as polyethylene glycol (PEG), reduced ROS production and the formation of FBGCs in vitro and in vivo [21].

However, it is important to note that the effectiveness of antioxidants in preventing FBGC formation may depend on several factors, such as the type and concentration of antioxidant used, the characteristics of the graft material, and the specific immune response of the host [12, 22]. Additionally, the use of antioxidants may also have potential drawbacks, such as interfering with the normal immune response to the graft material or affecting other cellular functions [23, 24]. Therefore, while incorporating antioxidants into a graft material may be a promising approach to reduce FBGC formation, further research is needed to determine the optimal conditions for their use and to fully understand their potential benefits and risks.

Silk fibroin is a natural macromolecule and degraded by proteolysis when it is implanted into the body [25]. Many FBGCs are observed around silk fibroin-based graft (Fig. 7.2). Interestingly, 4HR-incorporated silk fibroin graft shows less FBGC formation [26]. In addition, 4HR inhibits IL4-induced FBGC formation. 4HR inhibited diacylglycerol kinase-δ (DAGKδ) expression dose dependently, which is reflected and increased diacylglycerol (DAG) and decreased phosphatidic acid (PA) production in cells [26]. DAGKδ is an enzyme that phosphorylates DAG, converting it into phosphatidic acid (PA) and thereby reducing the intracellular levels of DAG [27].

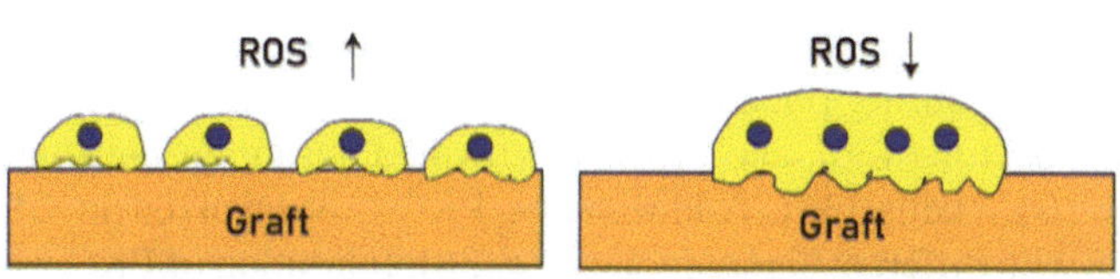

Fig. 7.1 The degradation of macromolecules requires the presence of numerous macrophages. During this process, energy is produced by mitochondria, which may lead to excessive production of reactive oxygen species (ROS). To counteract ROS-mediated apoptotic stress, macrophages fuse with one another, resulting in the formation of multinucleated cells. This fusion reduces the overall number of mitochondria and subsequently lowers ROS levels. However, the biodegrading ability of the multinucleated cell is lower than that of the sum of its individual macrophages

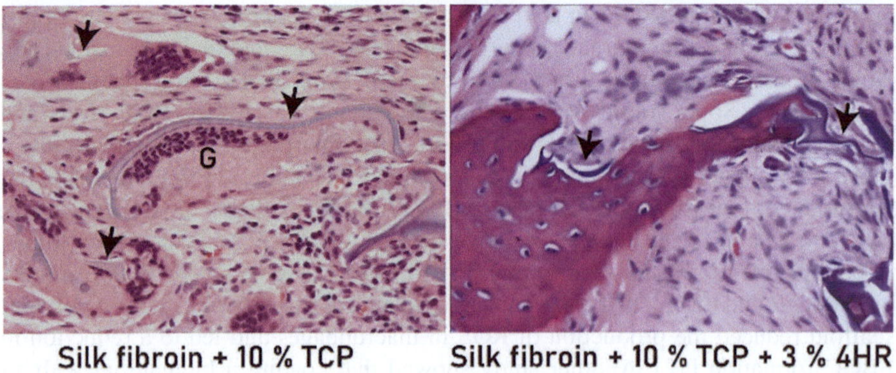

Fig. 7.2 The comparison between 4HR-incorporated silk graft and silk graft. At 8 weeks postoperation, the incorporation of 4HR in silk grafts was compared to silk grafts alone. In the silk fibroin +10% β-tricalcium phosphate group, multinucleated giant cells (G) were observed around the silk fibers (indicated by arrows). However, in the 4HR-incorporated group, the remnants of silk fibers were minimal, and new bone formation was evident. Additionally, the number of multinucleated giant cells observed in the 4HR-incorporated group was significantly reduced

DAG is an important lipid signaling molecule that is involved in the regulation of various cellular processes, including the activation of protein kinase C (PKC) and the production of ROS [28]. DAG levels are maintained as low levels in macrophages at resting conditions [29]. PKC is known to activate the NADPH oxidase complex, which is responsible for the production of ROS in macrophages [30]. PKC can activate a variety of proteolytic enzymes, such as matrix metalloproteinases (MMPs), cathepsins, and serine proteases, which are involved in tissue remodeling, antigen presentation, and host defense mechanisms [31]. Studies have shown that the activation of PKC can increase the expression and activity of MMPs and cathepsins in macrophages, leading to enhanced proteolytic activity [32, 33]. Furthermore, PKC activation can also increase the expression and release of cytokines and chemokines, which can further enhance the recruitment and activation of macrophages in tissues [34]. Interestingly, 4HR-incorporated silk fibroin graft shows fast biodegradation during its grafting [26].

PKC can be categorized into three groups based on their dependency on DAG and calcium. PKCδ is DAG-dependent but calcium-independent, while PKCζ is independent of both calcium and DAG [35]. Previous studies have investigated the activation of PKC during phagocytosis, revealing that PKC plays a role in FcR-mediated phagocytosis [36], and PKCδ is activated during IgG-mediated phagocytosis in Raw264.7 cells [37]. Additionally, PKC-ζ is involved in CR3-mediated phagocytosis with different signal molecules [38]. Inhibition of PKC with inhibitors has been shown to inhibit FcR and CR3-mediated phagocytosis in macrophages and monocytes [39, 40]. Therefore, studying the changes in phosphorylation levels of PKCδ and PKCζ after 4HR administration would be of interest.

Our unpublished findings show that administration of 10 μg/mL 4HR increases the phosphorylation levels of PKCδ and PKCζ at 8 h and decreases them at 24 h after administration (Fig. 7.3). PKC is synthesized as an inactive form and changes into a phospho-form and mature form upon activation, with different molecular weights depending on the type [41, 42]. Thus, the influence of 4HR on the cellular concentration of PKC and its activation can induce changes in the form of PKC.

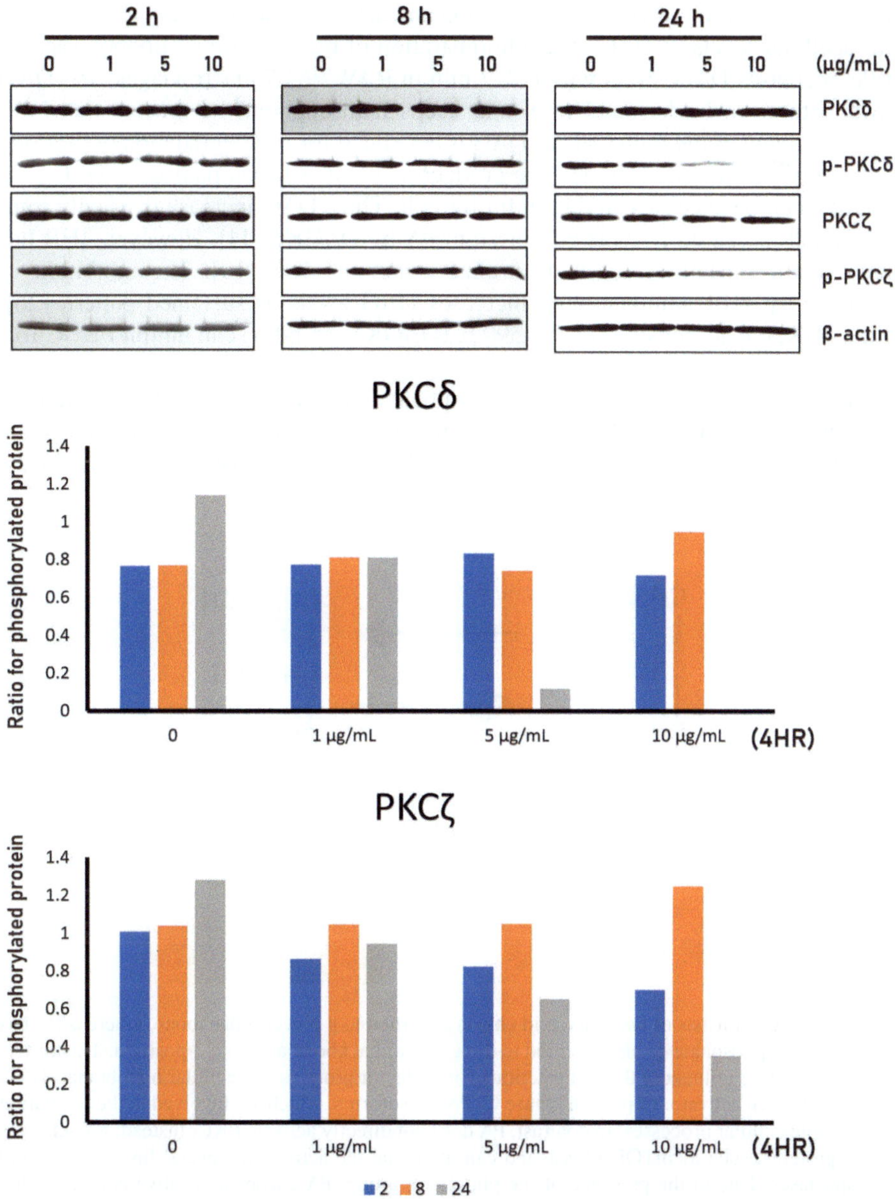

Fig. 7.3 After administration of 4HR, the expression levels of PKCδ, PKCζ, and their phosphorylated forms were evaluated. When treated with 10 μg/mL of 4HR, the ratio between the phosphorylated form and total protein increased at 8 h and decreased at 24 h for both PKCδ and PKCζ

Several studies have shown that the expression level and activity of DAGKδ are tightly regulated in response to changes in intracellular DAG levels [39]. For example, increased DAG levels can lead to the upregulation of DAGKδ expression and activity, which results in the conversion of DAG into PA and a decrease in the intracellular levels of DAG (Fig. 7.4). Conversely, decreased DAG levels can result in the downregulation of DAGKδ expression and activity, leading to an increase in the intracellular levels of DAG. The administration of bacterial toxin, lipopolysaccharide, increases DAG levels within 2–3 min in RAW 264.7 macrophages, and DAG level returns to background level and keeps it throughout the time course [43]. Though maintaining high level of DAG is beneficial for fast degradation of graft via activating proteolytic enzymes, the production of ROS accompanied by DAG production can be excessive and harmful for cell. Thus, DAG increase is usually transient, and increased DAG is converted to PA by DAGKδ [44]. However, 4HR has antioxidant capacity and can neutralize excessive ROS [10]. The inhibition of DAGKδ by 4HR administration increases DAG levels as sustained pattern [26]. Like 4HR, the administration of R59022 (DAGKδ inhibitor) can inhibit FBGC formation, too [22].

The incorporation of tri-calcium phosphate and 4HR with silk fibroin results in less intense FBGC formation compared to silk fibroin with tri-calcium phosphate alone [26] (Fig. 7.2). This suggests that 4HR may inhibit FBGC formation in the

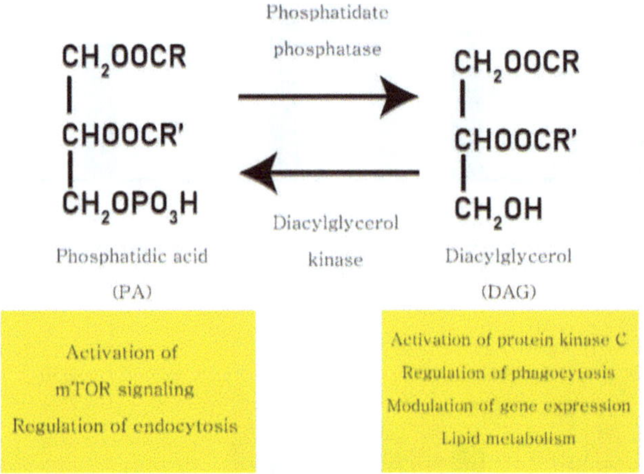

Fig. 7.4 DAG consists of two fatty acid chains esterified to a glycerol backbone, whereas PA has an additional phosphate group esterified to the glycerol backbone at the sn-3 position. This difference in structure influences their interactions with effector proteins and cellular membranes. DAG is a well-known activator of protein kinase C (PKC) isoforms, which are involved in the regulation of multiple cellular processes. In contrast, PA does not directly activate PKC. Instead, PA activates other proteins, such as mTOR kinase and can modulate the activity of several lipid kinases and phosphatases. Due to the presence of the phosphate group, PA carries a negative charge, which allows it to interact with positively charged amino acid residues in target proteins. In contrast, DAG lacks this charge and interacts with proteins through a different mechanism, mainly hydrophobic interactions

graft, and the incorporation of 4HR leads to more rapid biodegradation compared to grafts without 4HR. In vivo observations by McNally and Anderson [45] showed that vitamin E-modified poly(etherurethane) led to decreased biomaterial degradation coupled with increased FBGC formation.

Macrophages play a crucial role in clearing foreign materials implanted in the body, primarily through phagocytosis and degradation. During this process, macrophages increase metabolic activity, leading to the production of ROS and apoptotic stress [46, 47]. To counteract this stress, pro-survival pathways need to be activated, and phagocytic activity decreased [48]. One such strategy for cell survival is cell-to-cell fusion, which results in decreased phagocytic activity. Crohn's disease patients' macrophages have a higher fusion index, reduced cell function, and low phagocytic activity [49]. Enzymes such as PA and DAGK regulate the pro-survival pathway and inflammatory reaction [50]. Therefore, understanding macrophages' role and associated pathways is crucial for successful biomaterial grafting.

7.2 Regeneration of Vessel

The damage of major vessel and its reconstruction are important issue in the tissue engineering. There are various types of alloplastic materials used in vascular reconstruction.

1. Synthetic grafts: These are made of materials such as Dacron or PTFE (polytetrafluoroethylene) and are often used in large vessel reconstructions.
2. Biologic grafts: These are derived from human or animal tissue, such as veins or arteries, and are often used in smaller vessel reconstructions.
3. Collagen-based materials: These are derived from collagen and are often used to support tissue regeneration.
4. Tissue-engineered materials: These are created using cells and biomaterials to create a living replacement tissue.

These materials have several limitations.

1. Risk of infection: Synthetic grafts can be susceptible to infection, which can be difficult to treat and may result in the need for removal of the graft.
2. Limited durability: Synthetic grafts can be subject to wear and tear over time, which can lead to graft failure or other complications.
3. Risk of thrombosis: Synthetic grafts can be prone to thrombosis (blood clots), which can lead to graft occlusion and subsequent failure.
4. Immune response: Alloplastic materials can trigger an immune response, which can lead to rejection or other complications.
5. Technical challenges: Vascular reconstruction using alloplastic materials can be technically challenging, requiring specialized skills and expertise.

In synthetic grafts, the risk of thrombosis can be attributed to factors such as the graft's porosity, surface properties, and diameter [51]. Smaller diameter grafts are more prone to thrombosis because they have a higher surface-area-to-volume ratio, which can promote clotting. Surface properties, such as roughness or coating, can also affect the graft's thrombogenicity [52]. In addition, the immune response can manifest as a foreign body reaction, which is characterized by the infiltration of inflammatory cells and the formation of scar tissue around the graft [53]. This reaction can lead to the narrowing or occlusion of the graft, reducing blood flow and potentially leading to graft failure.

Bioactive molecule preventing thrombosis has been included in artificial vessel. One such molecule is heparin, a naturally occurring anticoagulant that inhibits blood clotting by binding to and activating antithrombin III, a protein that blocks the action of clotting factors in the blood [54]. Heparin can be coated onto the surface of artificial blood vessels to prevent thrombosis [55].

Other bioactive molecules that have been studied for their potential to prevent thrombosis include prostacyclin (PGI2), nitric oxide (NO), and tissue plasminogen activator (tPA) [56]. PGI2 is a vasodilator and inhibitor of platelet aggregation, while NO is a potent vasodilator and inhibitor of platelet activation and adhesion [56]. tPA is an enzyme that activates the conversion of plasminogen to plasmin, which dissolves blood clots [56]. These molecules can also be coated onto the surface of artificial blood vessels to prevent thrombosis. However, there has been no paper that mentions coating these molecules onto the surface of artificial blood vessels.

Spirulinas maxima (SP) extract is a natural antithrombogenic material that has been used in various experiments [57, 58]. Therefore, an artificial vessel with a surface that prevents acute thrombosis may be successful without requiring ex-vivo cell culture. In histological analysis, the luminal surface of SP-incorporated silk vessel is found to be fully lined with endothelial cells, and thrombosis is not observed (Fig. 7.5). This may be attributed to the presence of SP extract in the silk fibroin matrix. The middle layer of the artificial vessel showed regenerated collagen fibers in a special stain (data not shown), and numerous fibroblasts were observed in the middle and outer layers [59].

The silk mat obtained from silk cocoon exhibits several desirable biological and mechanical properties, making it a suitable material for use as a vascular patch [60]. The manufacturing process of silk mat is relatively simple and cost-effective, involving peeling of the silk cocoon [60]. In comparison to the SF vascular patch [61], the silk mat is easier to manufacture. For use as a vascular patch, the material should possess sufficient mechanical strength to withstand suture retention [62]. Previous research has demonstrated that under wet conditions, the silk mat exhibits the highest tensile strength when compared to collagen and PTFE membranes [63]. Furthermore, it displays superior suture retention strength in comparison to collagen [60]. The 4HR-incorporated silk patch can be successfully applied to a carotid artery defect and sutured to the arterial wall without tearing in wet conditions [64].

Silk obtained from silkworms is composed of two main components—fibroin and sericin [65]. The fibroin forms the core of the silk filament [66], while the sericin is attached to the fibroin fibers and serves to bind them together [67]. During patch angioplasty, there is no excessive blood leakage observed in any of the groups (direct closure, PTFE patch, and 4HR-incorporated silk patch), and angiography

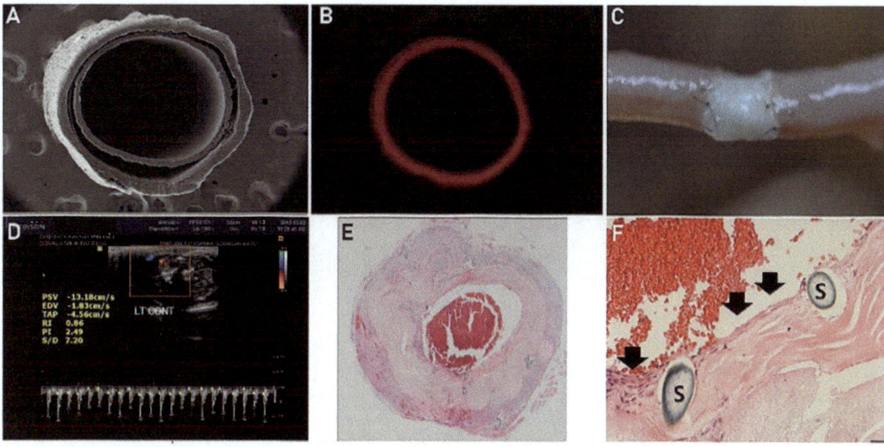

Fig. 7.5 Silk fibroin/ poly-caprolactone/SP extract-based artificial vessel. (**a**) Scanning electron image of multilayered artificial vessel. (**b**) SP extract showed bright red color in fluorescent microscopic image. (**c**) The artificial vessel was anastomosed to the end of carotid artery. (**d**) Doppler image showed successful functioning of grafted vessel. (**e**) Cells were grown into the artificial vessel. (**f**) The endothelial cells (arrows) were regenerated. Nylon suture (S) used for vessel connection was also observed (modified from authors' previous publication [59])

confirmed artery patency [64]. However, in the PTFE patch group, minor blood leakage is observed around the patch after the vascular operation [64]. In contrast, the 4HR silk patch group exhibited less blood leakage and better adhesion to the artery wall than the PTFE patch group [64]. The sericin protein, which acts as a bonding agent [67], may have played a role in enhancing the attachment of the silk patch to the vessel.

It has been found that patch angioplasty is more effective than primary closure in reducing the likelihood of stroke and restenosis [68]. Primary closure of small-diameter carotid arteries following endarterectomy can lead to compromised blood flow and a higher risk of postoperative restenosis [69, 70]. In our research [64], angiographic analysis showed that the arterial diameter in the control group was significantly decreased after direct closure. However, in the 4HR silk and PTFE groups, there was no considerable reduction in diameter, and stability was maintained (Fig. 7.6).

Ultrasonographic assessment confirmed that the 4HR-silk and PTFE groups experienced more favorable blood flow [64]. The ultrasound results showed a notable difference in blood flow velocity between the direct closure group and the other groups ($p < 0.05$). This suggests that a reduced artery diameter in the direct closure group led to increased blood flow velocity in the affected area [64]. On the other hand, angiographic examination revealed that the 4HR silk and PTFE groups experienced no significant changes in blood flow velocity post-angioplasty [64]. These results suggest that patch angioplasty is a more effective technique for repairing artery wall defects than direct closure, and that the 4HR silk patch material is comparable in efficacy to the commercial PTFE patch product.

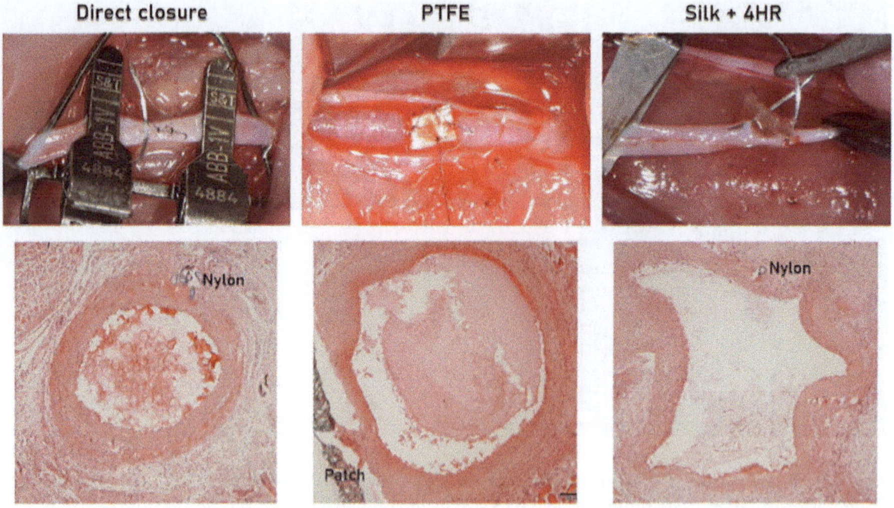

Fig. 7.6 Implementation of the vascular patch in a carotid artery defect model. The cross-sectional area was significantly larger in the PTFE and silk+4HR groups compared to the direct closure group. While the nonbiodegradable PTFE patch was visible in the histological section, the silk+4HR patch was not detected around the nylon suture, which was utilized for silk+4HR patch fixation

Previous studies have indicated that 4HR can hinder foreign body reactions and the development of giant cells surrounding graft materials [26]. This is achieved through the suppression of DAGK within macrophages. Furthermore, 4HR aids in the biodegradation process of graft materials, ultimately promoting healing and regeneration in soft tissues [26, 71]. Additionally, 4HR has been observed to inhibit the expression of tumor necrosis factor-α (TNF-α) in raw cells, thereby facilitating rapid epithelization and collagen regeneration in burn wounds [72]. We observed no inflammatory or immunological reactions in the 4HR silk group, but instead, we noted the regeneration of endothelial tissue in the silk patch area [64]. In summary, our findings suggest that the incorporation of 4HR into the silk patch is effective in reducing immune reaction and promoting endothelium regeneration, thereby contributing to the success of the silk patch angioplasty.

7.3 The Surface Treatment of Dental Implant

The use of dental implants has become widespread for replacing missing teeth. Depending on the implant design, the upper part of the fixture may protrude into the oral mucosa. As every implant is structured to mimic the tooth crown, a certain portion of it must remain uncovered with biological barriers like the mucosa. Unfortunately, the oral cavity is home to various types of bacteria, and the exposed surface of the implant can serve as a site for bacterial adhesion, leading to inflammation. While some implant failures result from the mechanical properties of the implant itself, the majority of failures stem from peri-implant inflammation [73].

Successful osseointegration of dental implants relies heavily on rapid bone regeneration around the fixture, which primarily faces the alveolar bone. However, healing capacity varies widely among individuals, and systemic diseases like diabetes mellitus and osteoporosis can adversely affect the success rate of the implant [74]. To encourage rapid bone regeneration, surface modifications have been made to dental implants, with the goal of increasing surface roughness to enhance cellular attachment [75]. This, in turn, can lead to an increase in alkaline phosphatase activity [76]. However, rough surfaces can also provide a site for bacteria to adhere more easily than smooth surfaces [77], and they can be more difficult to clean thoroughly. For this reason, some dental implants have highly polished surfaces around the neck of the fixture [78].

Rather than relying on a rough surface to accelerate new bone formation, some dental implants can be coated with bioactive molecules. One such molecule is hydroxyapatite (HA), which is the main component of bones and has been used as a graft material [79]. Dental implants coated with HA have also been developed and utilized for this purpose. However, HA-coated implants have frequently failed in ophthalmology applications due to infection [80, 81]. This is because HA is highly hydrophilic and provides a favorable site for bacterial adhesion [82, 83].

The success rate of HA-coated dental implants has been a topic of some controversy. While many reports have indicated a high success rate for these implants [84, 85], negative findings have also emerged from long-term follow-up studies [86]. A recent study directly comparing different dental implants uncovered that those with HA coatings tend to experience increased failure rates when the surface is exposed to the oral environment [87]. Considering HA's excellent biocompatibility and its ability to promote swift osseointegration in low-quality bone, creating an infection-resistant HA coating could hold significant potential for clinical use.

4HR is a recognized antiseptic [88] that exhibits no toxic effects at concentrations up to 50 μg/ml in Caco-2 cells [89]. However, due to its organic nature, 4HR is sensitive to heat treatment, which poses challenges in creating an antimicrobial coating with HA on metal surfaces. If this process can be accomplished at room temperature, it is possible to coat HA with 4HR onto metallic surfaces without affecting their biological properties.

To overcome this challenge, researchers utilized an aerosol deposition system as detailed in other sources [90]. The process began by dissolving 4HR in ethanol, followed by vigorously mixing HA powder with the 4HR ethanol solution for an hour. The ethanol was subsequently evaporated using a rotary evaporator, yielding a HA-4HR blended powder. This mixture was placed in a vibrating aerosol chamber containing fine airborne particles, which were then propelled by oxygen gas onto the titanium disk or implant within the deposition chamber (Fig. 7.7). The chamber was continuously evacuated with the aid of mechanical booster and rotary pumps. Particles were released from the nozzle with a slit-type opening (0.5 mm × 25.4 mm), while the motorized stage containing the titanium disk or implant moved perpendicularly to the slit-type opening's length. By scanning the motorized stage,

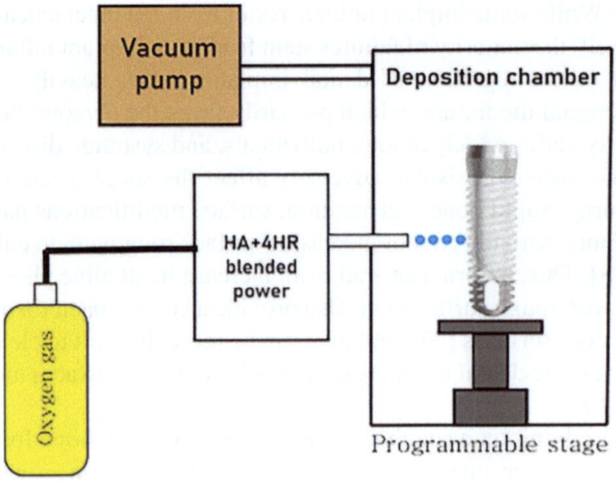

Fig. 7.7 Schematic drawing for aerosol deposition technique

researchers were able to deposit a 5 μm thick coating onto the titanium disc or implant. The final HA coating exhibited a stoichiometric Ca/P ratio of 1.67.

The HA-coated surface is susceptible to biofilm formation by microorganisms, which can lead to inflammation around the implant fixture. To address this, a combination of HA particles and 4HR was coated on a titanium surface [91]. The HA + 4HR combination coating showed clear advantages over the HA coating alone in this study. Firstly, it had better cellular attachment. Secondly, it had higher expression of osteocalcin and alkaline phosphatase activity than the HA coating alone. Thirdly, in the presence of infection, the HA + 4HR coating had a higher removal torque value, bone formation value, and bone-to-implant contact value than the HA coating alone.

The X-ray diffraction (XRD) pattern of the titanium surface coated with HA displayed peaks originating from both the coating and the substrate [91]. The diffraction pattern of the coated layer aligned well with the hexagonal phase of stoichiometric HA (ICDD, 086–0740). However, the relatively high peak intensity from the titanium indicated a thin HA film thickness. When 4HR was added to the HA film, the HA diffraction pattern remained unaltered. No peaks were observed from potential by-products such as calcite, β-tri-calcium phosphate, calcium oxide, or calcium nitrate, signifying a high-quality crystalline phase for the deposited HA film.

The infrared absorption spectrum of the HA displayed characteristic vibrational modes (Fig. 7.8). The HA + 4HR coating exhibited strong absorption peaks consistent with the recognized stretching and bending modes of $-CH_2-$ in an aliphatic hydrocarbon. Through the XRD and FT-IR patterns, it was verified that the HA + 4HR coating was successfully applied to the titanium surface [91].

4HR is a well-known antiseptic that has been utilized as an ingredient in oral gargling solutions. It was historically used as a therapeutic drug for infectious

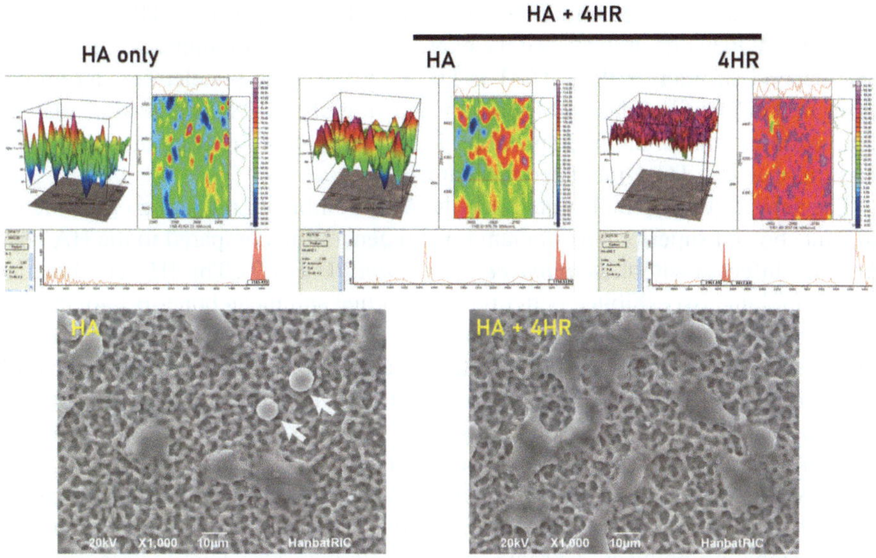

Fig. 7.8 Distribution of FT-IR spectra for HA and 4HR (top row). HA and 4HR demonstrate uniform distribution on the titanium plate surface. Upon seeding MG63 cells on each disc, the HA group exhibits inadequate cell attachment (indicated by arrows) after 4 h. In contrast, the HA + 4HR group reveals well-dispersed cells at the 4-h mark following initial seeding

diseases and has been consumed by humans in olive oil without any reported complications [92, 93]. Due to its hydrophobic nature, a direct drug release behavior curve could not be generated in this study. However, the calcium release behavior curve of the HA coating, using the same method as this study, has already been published [94]. As HA degrades, 4HR in HA will be released. Interestingly, the HA disc also demonstrated antimicrobial properties against *S. aureus* and *P. intermedia* [91], likely due to the release of free calcium ion from the coated surface [94]. Free calcium ion is known to be toxic to certain bacterial species [95, 96]. While the HA coating did not produce a *P. gingivalis* inhibitory zone, the 4HR combination coating did. This suggests that the 4HR combination coating has a more favorable antibacterial spectrum when compared to the HA coating alone [91].

Cellular attachment was evaluated at 1, 4, and 24 h after MG63 cell seeding onto the coated disc. The combination coating of HA with 4HR showed a faster and more extensive cellular attachment than the HA coating alone (Fig. 7.8). Consequently, upregulation of ALP activity and osteocalcin expression was observed [91]. While the early attachment of MG63 cells to the 4HR combination coating could activate the cells, the mechanism of rapid attachment and spreading remains unclear. It has been reported that 4HR can induce intracellular calcium influx in various types of cells, leading to changes in the permeability of ions and ionic homeostasis [96]. Additionally, intracellular calcium content can be modified by bacterial lipids, including those generated under the influence of 4HR [97]. When 4HR was administered to MG63 cells, it increased the expression of transglutaminase-1 (TG-1) in a dose-dependent manner [91]. TG-1 is known to promote platelet-derived growth factor-dependent fibroblast proliferation and migration [98], suggesting that the rapid cellular attachment and spreading induced by the 4HR combination coating might be due to a TG-1-mediated mechanism.

The animal study demonstrated that the 4HR combination coating on the dental implant showed superior peri-implant bone regeneration compared to the HA coating when infected with *A. actinomycetemcomitans* (Fig. 7.9). The 4HR combination coated implant also exhibited better removal torque and mean bone-to-implant contact compared to the HA-coated implant [91]. The reasons for the enhanced bone regeneration around the 4HR combination coated implant can be explained as follows. Firstly, 4HR, being an antiseptic agent, was more effective in an infection state compared to HA alone. Secondly, 4HR may have promoted cellular attachment to the implant surface, as observed in the in vitro experiment. Thirdly, 4HR can affect the regulation of NF-kB functions, which are involved in osteoclastogenesis [99]. This may impair osteoclastogenesis by disrupting the RANK-mediated NF-kB signaling pathway. Chronic use of 4HR may also lead to osteosclerosis [100], which could be attributed to impaired osteoclastogenesis.

In conclusion, dental implants face challenges such as bacterial adhesion and varying individual healing capacities. To address these issues, the combination of HA particles and 4HR was coated on titanium surfaces, resulting in improved cellular attachment, increased osteocalcin and alkaline phosphatase activity, and enhanced bone formation and bone-to-implant contact values compared to HA coatings alone. The promising outcomes of the HA + 4HR combination coating suggest its potential to enhance dental implant success, particularly in the presence of infection, offering a valuable advancement in dental implant technology.

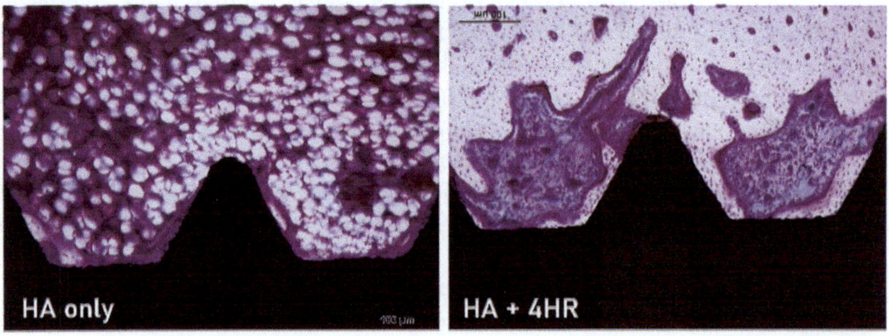

Fig. 7.9 Histological analysis of implant therapy. Prior to placement, both HA and HA + 4HR implants exhibited bacterial contamination. Eight weeks after surgery, the HA + 4HR group displayed a significantly greater amount of new bone formation compared to the HA-only group (scale bar = 100 μm)

7.4 Biodegradable Silk Suture

The use of suture materials is widespread in the surgical field, and the suture market has seen annual increases in millions of dollars [101, 102]. The purpose of suture material is to aid in the natural healing process by closing off wounded areas, and therefore, an ideal suture material must possess both proper biological compatibility and physical strength [103]. Sutures can be classified as absorbable or non-absorbable, with non-absorbable sutures requiring removal, which can be a challenge in certain clinical situations [104]. In such cases, biodegradable sutures are recommended.

Silk suture, composed of silk fibroin protein from *Bombyx mori* and coating material, is considered nonbiodegradable because it takes approximately 2 years to fully degrade [65]. Despite being a relatively inexpensive material, silk suture is prone to inflammation caused by microorganisms that can attach to it [104]. To address this issue, antibiotics have been incorporated into silk suture [104]. However, there are currently no reports of biodegradable silk suture with antimicrobial properties.

4HR, an amphiphilic molecule with hydrophobic and hydrophilic properties, has been used as an antiseptic [92] and food ingredient [105]. By interacting with target proteins via both hydrophobic and hydrophilic interactions, 4HR can be incorporated into proteins such as silk fibroin. 4HR-incorporated silk scaffold has been shown to have improved ability as a bone graft material or membrane for guided bone regeneration [106, 107]. Recent research has demonstrated that 4HR-incorporated silk scaffold reduces foreign body reaction and accelerates graft degradation [26].

Many synthetic suture materials are degraded mainly by hydrolysis [108], while natural polymers such as collagen suture are degraded by proteolysis [109]. A group of matrix metalloproteinases (MMPs) can degrade silk fibroin [28], and MMPs are highly expressed during acute inflammatory and late remodeling phases [110]. MMPs are mainly produced by monocytes and macrophages [111], and it was unclear whether 4HR can increase the expression of MMPs in macrophages. If so, 4HR-incorporated silk suture can be degraded according to the time schedule of macrophage activation during the wound healing process.

4HR, due to its hydrophobic long alkyl group and low solubility in water [112], can easily be incorporated into hydrophobic domains of biological molecules [113]. As silk fibroin is mainly composed of hydrophobic domains [104], 4HR can be easily incorporated into silk suture materials when the proper media is selected. In our study, commercially available silk suture materials are treated with 4HR, and successful incorporation was examined using FT-IR spectra [9]. The FT-IR spectra show that silk suture treated with 4HR has enhanced relative absorption of protein and a significantly increased amide III peak corresponding to the β-sheet conformation (Fig. 7.10). However, the physical strength of the silk suture is not weakened by the treatment, and the knot-holding capacity is improved (Fig. 7.10). Additionally, 4HR-incorporated silk suture demonstrated antimicrobial properties [9].

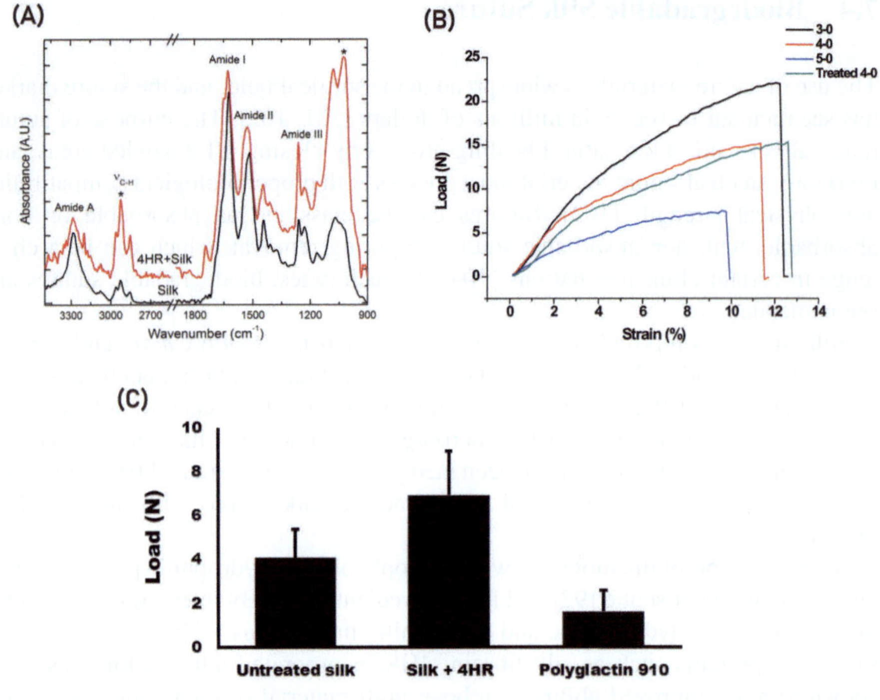

Fig. 7.10 Properties of 4HR-treated silk sutures. (**a**) FT-IR spectra show similar amide peaks for untreated and 4HR-treated silk, with minor alterations and enhanced β-sheet conformation in 4HR-treated silk. (**b**) Stress-strain curve indicates increased physical strength with larger suture diameter; 4HR-treated 4–0 sutures have similar yield strength and higher strain compared to untreated sutures. (**c**) 4HR-treated sutures display the highest knot-holding capacity among 4–0 sutures

4HR has been shown to enter the nucleus of cells and influence gene expression [114], as well as incorporate into the hydrophobic domain of proteins and affect their function [113]. It was hypothesized that the action of MMPs, a group of proteolytic enzymes responsible for degrading extracellular matrix proteins, may be regulated by 4HR administration due to its ability to modulate the NF-kB signaling pathway [115]. In subsequent research, 4HR has been identified as a potent stimulator of TGF-β1 [106], and the expression levels of MMPs are regulated by TGF-β1 [116]. Macrophages are treated with 4HR, and higher expression of MMP-2, −3, and − 9 is observed compared to untreated controls [9]. The proteolysis of silk fibroin protein by MMP-2, −3, and − 9 is demonstrated, with MMP-2 being the most efficient [9]. Mechanical strength measurements show that the 4HR-incorporated silk suture has lower mechanical strength after MMPs treatment compared to untreated silk suture, demonstrating that 4HR increases MMP activity [9].

In animal experiments, silk suture, 4HR-treated silk suture, and polyglactin 910 were implanted under the skin of rats [9]. Gradual volume loss of grafts is observed in both the 4HR-treated silk suture and polyglactin 910 groups until 11 weeks after implantation, with a faster rate of volume loss observed in sonography starting at

9 weeks after implantation [9]. The expression of MMPs was not high in the untreated silk and 4HR-treated silk groups at 4 weeks and 8 weeks after implantation [9]. However, the 4HR-treated silk suture showed a similar level of biodegradation compared to polyglactin 910 suture, demonstrating its potential as a biodegradable suture material [9] (Fig. 7.11).

In conclusion, this study demonstrated that 4HR, a resorcinolic lipid, can be successfully incorporated into silk suture materials without weakening their physical strength or knot-holding capacity. The 4HR-incorporated silk suture also demonstrated antimicrobial properties, which is a beneficial characteristic in clinical practice. Additionally, the study showed that 4HR can increase the expression of MMPs in macrophages, leading to accelerated biodegradation of the silk suture material. Animal experiments further demonstrated the biodegradable properties of the 4HR-treated silk suture. Overall, this study provides insight into the potential of 4HR-incorporated silk suture as a biomaterial for use in surgical procedures.

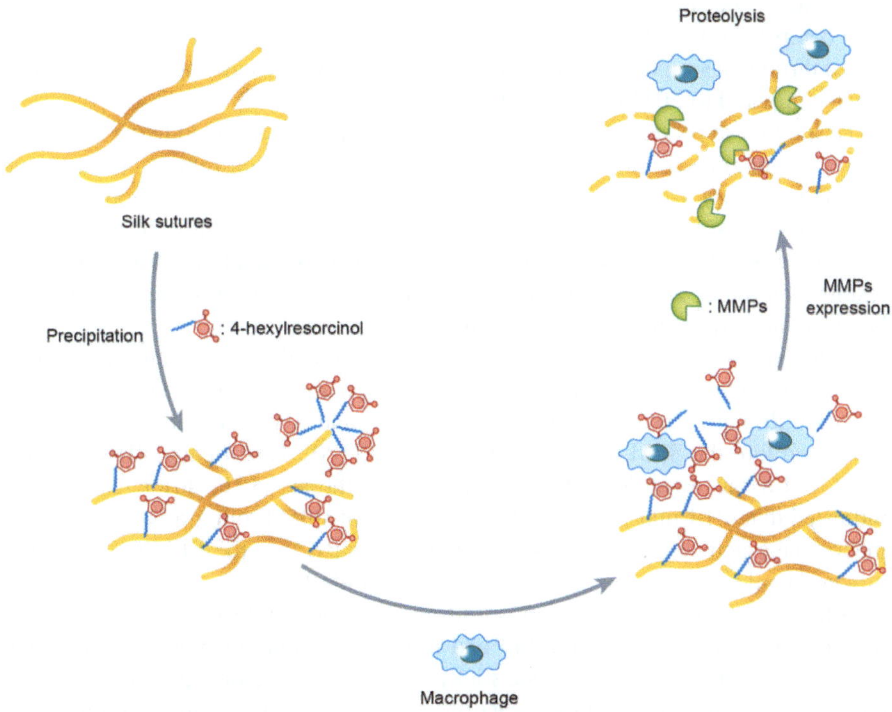

Fig. 7.11 Hypothesized mechanism for suture degradation aided by 4HR. As an amphiphilic compound, 4HR has both hydrophobic and hydrophilic regions. Its hydrophobic long alkyl group interacts with silk sutures' hydrophobic domains. To engage with the hydrophilic domain, 4HR outcompetes water, forming high-density micelles near the suture's hydrophilic domain through preferential hydration. Most of these micelles are released rapidly after implantation, as 4HR's hydrogen bond with silk protein is weaker than with water. During wound remodeling, firmly bound 4HR in hydrophobic domains is exposed by macrophages, which then release 4HR, inducing MMPs production to digest silk suture material (reproduced from author's previous publication [9])

7.5 Bone Graft and Guided Bone Regeneration

7.5.1 Membrane for Guided Bone Regeneration

The primary objective of incorporating a barrier membrane in guided bone regeneration (GBR) is to preserve adequate space for future bone growth [117]. In dental practice, absorbable collagen membranes or non-absorbable expanded polytetrafluoroethlene (ePTFE) membranes have traditionally been employed for GBR [118]. However, due to their high cost, their application in clinical settings is restricted despite their demonstrated efficacy in bone regeneration.

To address this cost issue, researchers have turned their attention toward silk fiber as a possible material for barrier membranes [118]. Prior investigations have shown that silk-based barrier membranes could promote bone regeneration in animal models. The use of silk fibroin film generated by casting method, for instance, was found to be superior in terms of bone regeneration when compared to uncovered controls [119, 120]. Similarly, the silkworm cocoon membrane, which is produced through a simple separation process, showed better bone regeneration results when compared to ePTFE membrane [63].

Despite these promising findings, there are some limitations to using silk-based barrier membranes. Firstly, they are non-absorbable, and their removal through surgery is necessary after the desired bone formation is achieved. Previous research also noted the silk fibroin film's high fragility and low operability during surgery [119, 120]. While the silkworm cocoon membrane exhibited better bone formation results than the ePTFE membrane [63], mechanical separation of the cocoon could be labor-intensive and difficult to automate.

In this investigation, we assessed the efficacy of a silk fabric membrane (SFM) as an alternative silk-based barrier membrane in an animal model. The SFM is fabricated utilizing a textile production technique, and 4HR, an antiseptic agent, is integrated into the SFM to enable drug delivery [120]. Historically, 4HR has been employed as an ingredient in lozenges for sore throats [121]. Prior research has indicated that 4HR may facilitate the breakdown of silk fibroin grafts by promoting macrophage activation [26]. The researchers posited that the SFM's degradation process would be hastened through the release of 4HR.

Silk fiber consists of two proteins: fibroin and sericin. Fibroin serves as the main protein, exhibiting biocompatibility and minimal immune response in the human body [122]. Conversely, sericin is a sticky protein that envelops fibroin. While sericin is generally regarded as biocompatible, there have been accounts of immune and irritation reactions associated with it [123, 124]. In the current research, silk sericin was eliminated via a degumming procedure to produce the SFM.

The traditional SFM exhibited a gentle and smooth surface with an ivory hue [107]. Its primary benefit is the capacity for mass production with consistent quality and affordability. In clinical applications, it can be used for bone defects ranging from small to large, and the membrane's form can be effortlessly altered using scissors. Nevertheless, due to the high molecular weight and crystallinity of natural silk material, the conventional SFM's lack of rigidity and non-absorbable characteristics require a follow-up surgery for removal. In our previous study, both the 4HR-integrated SFM group and the traditional SFM group displayed increased bone regeneration rates in comparison to the unshielded control group [107]. These results align with earlier investigations on various silk-based barrier membranes [119, 120]. The conventional SFM functions as a barrier membrane, impeding soft tissue ingrowth during the bone regeneration process [107].

Collagen membranes offer the benefit of progressive resorption during bone regeneration [125]. If incorporating 4HR allows for complete resorption of the silk membrane, a subsequent surgery for membrane removal would be redundant, as observed with collagen membranes. However, silk is typically regarded as non-absorbable [126]. Despite this, a few studies have proposed that silk fibroin may gradually degrade after a prolonged period in vivo [123]. Both in vivo and in vitro, silk fibroin can be incrementally degraded by proteolytic enzymes [127, 128]. Macrophages are crucial in the phagocytosis of foreign particles and the release of proteolytic enzymes [129]. 4HR has the potential to enhance macrophage activation by inhibiting foreign body giant cell formation within the silk fibroin graft [26].

In our previous research, the remaining membrane was more prevalent in the conventional SFM group compared to the 4HR-integrated SFM group (Fig. 7.12). This implies that the inclusion of 4HR expedites the partial breakdown of the SFM. For clinical significance, the SFM should be entirely absorbed. However, this study did not observe complete resorption [107]. Additional investigations involving extended healing durations and varying 4HR concentrations are required to assess the impact of 4HR on silk fibroin degradation.

In conclusion, silk-based barrier membranes have shown promising results in promoting bone regeneration, but their non-absorbable nature and fragility during surgery pose some limitations. We investigated the effectiveness of the SFM with and without the incorporation of the antiseptic agent 4HR in promoting bone regeneration [107]. Both SFM groups demonstrated higher bone regeneration rates than the uncovered control group, and there was no significant difference between the two SFM groups ($P > 0.05$). The addition of 4HR appeared to accelerate the partial degradation of the SFM, but further research is needed to determine if complete resorption can be achieved. The SFM has the advantage of being mass-produced at low cost with uniform quality and easy shaping. These findings suggest that SFM, with or without 4HR incorporation, may be a promising alternative to commercial barrier membranes in guided bone regeneration.

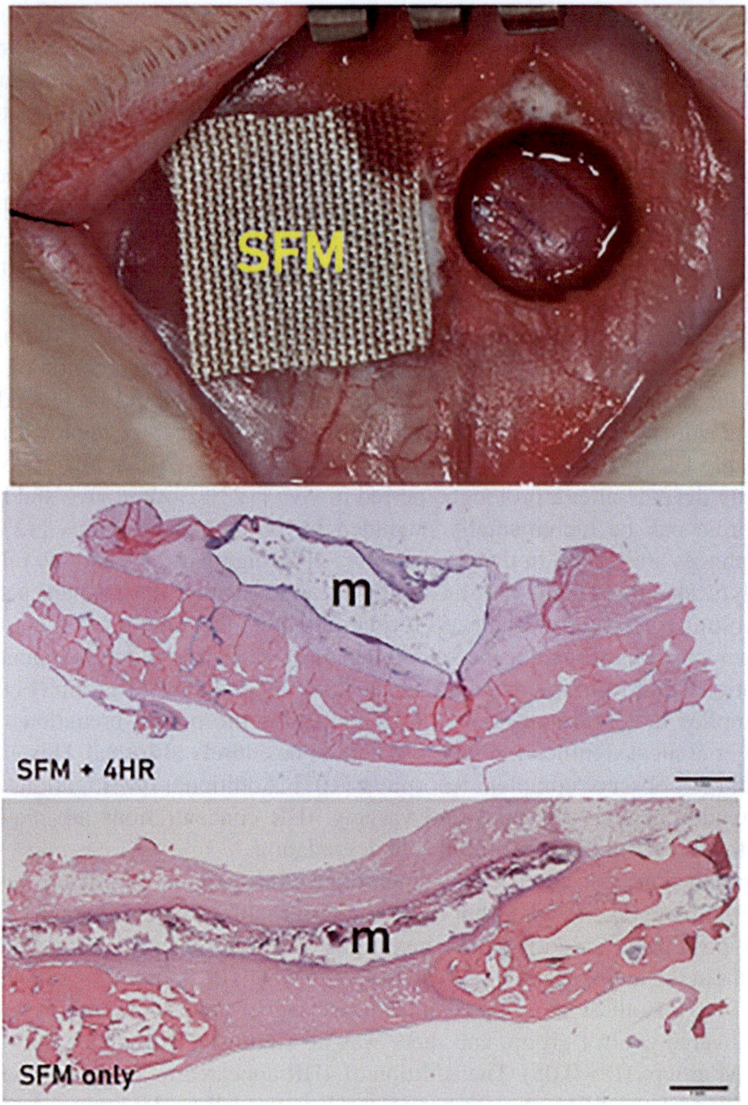

Fig. 7.12 Usage of silk fabric membrane (SFM) in a rabbit calvarial defect model (top). The SFM dimensions were 10 mm × 10 mm. Eight weeks' post-surgery, the SFM + 4HR group (middle) exhibited a considerably smaller residual SFM compared to the SFM-only group (bottom) (m: residual membrane)

7.5.2 Bone Graft

Bone defects in the field of oral and maxillofacial surgery often occur due to various causes such as trauma and tumours, resulting in the need for bone grafting. Although autologous bone is considered the most ideal material for reconstructing the defect area, there are issues related to complications at the donor site, limited harvesting volume, and resorption [130]. Therefore, numerous studies have been conducted to develop an ideal bone graft material that is convenient to use, unlimited in quantity, has adjustable absorption rates, and can easily restore the patient's condition aesthetically and functionally.

Our previous study attempted to create a more ideal bone graft material by adding 4HR to HA, which is currently the most preferred bone graft material [131]. We aimed to evaluate the bone regeneration capability of this new composite material in a rat model [131]. Two materials, HA and 4HR, were used in this experiment. HA has been traditionally preferred as an alternative to autologous bone grafts [132]. Some studies have reported that synthetic bone grafts may have lower bone healing rates, higher infection rates, and poorer mechanical alignment than autologous bone grafts in long-term follow-up [133]. Other studies have suggested that HA may need to be combined with other materials or growth factors to enhance its osteoconductive and osteoinductive properties [132]. We expected that if we could create a new compound without altering the characteristics of HA, the resulting new bone graft material would have excellent biocompatibility, adhere well to adjacent hard and soft tissues, and benefit from the advantages of 4HR.

The antimicrobial properties of 4HR were believed to contribute to infection resistance, while its ability to suppress osteoclast function [99] and its anti-inflammatory effects were thought to aid bone formation and reduce inflammatory responses in the graft host [8]. The scanning electron microscope (SEM) observations of HA and 4HR mixture showed that the two substances naturally fused together, forming a new starfish-shaped compound [131].

The new composite material showed superior bone formation during the initial 4 weeks compared to the group without the graft, based on the results of micro-computed tomography (micro-CT) analysis and histological analysis [131]. The reasons for this finding may include 4HR's ability to enhance cell attachment and its effects on osteoclast dysfunction, which promote bone formation. Previous research has reported that 4HR affects the regulation of NF-κB function [115], causing damage to the NF-κB signaling pathway mediated by the receptor activator of nuclear factor-kappa B and leading to osteoclast dysfunction [99]. At 8 weeks, there was no statistically significant difference in bone formation between the experimental and control groups, suggesting that the effects of 4HR on bone formation primarily occurred during the initial stages of bone regeneration [131]. Further research is needed to investigate the duration of 4HR's effects in vivo and to determine why its bone-forming ability did not persist until the eighth week.

We investigated the use of 4HR-incorporated porcine bone to enhance bone formation in a rat calvarial critical-sized bony defect model [134]. 4HR was successfully incorporated into porcine bone, demonstrating a steady release in vitro over 18 days [134]. The released 4HR suppressed the TNF-α-induced NF-kB signaling pathway, which in turn led to increased expression of bone formation marker proteins (Fig. 7.13). As a result, enhanced new bone formation was observed, making this the first report of successful new bone formation using 4HR-incorporated porcine bone graft material.

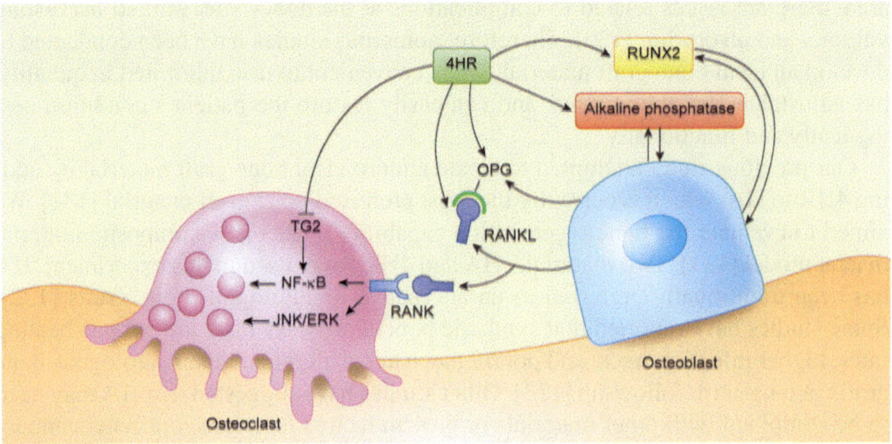

Fig. 7.13 The figure legend illustrates the effect of administering 4HR on the expression of runx2 and alkaline phosphatase, which are known to stimulate the activity of osteoblasts and promote new bone formation. In addition, 4HR administration inhibits transglutaminase-2 (TG2) activity and the NF-κB signaling pathway, leading to a reduction in osteoclast activity

In addition to porcine bone, the study examined the use of 4HR-treated bovine bone, acquired from a local grocery store, as a graft material [71]. After basic processing, this bone showed antibacterial properties and good cellular adhesion. However, the degradation rate of the 4HR-treated bovine bone was higher than that of the untreated control, and its rapid degradation velocity did not contribute to new bone regeneration. We suggest using a lower concentration of 4HR for bovine bone grafts in future studies to address this issue.

The control group in the study, treated with a 24-h ethanol wash, exhibited new bone deposition bordering the graft without inflammation [71]. This indicates that graft material processes originating from bovine bone may be a viable option for future investigations. The graft materials used in the study were sterilized by ethylene oxide, which did not reduce the osteoinductivity of bone morphogenetic proteins. The only unknown variable in this study was the concentration of 4HR in the graft. Future studies should determine the optimal 4HR concentration for bone grafts.

Apart from hydroxyapatite-based inorganic materials, natural proteins like sericin can also serve as osteoinduction materials when treated with 4HR [135]. Sericin, an industrial by-product, is produced during the degumming process, which can affect its conformation as it is an insect protein [10]. Grafted sericin may elicit various macrophage responses, primarily mediated by toll-like receptors (TLRs), which recognize foreign materials [136]. Foreign proteins with a β-sheet structure can activate TLR-2, leading macrophages to express BMP-2 [137]. Utilizing this feature in bone grafts could enhance new bone formation.

Upon treating p53 and silk fibroin with 4HR, the proportion of β-sheet structures in these proteins increases [9, 138]. Therefore, sericin is treated with 4HR and tested as a bone graft material. The 4HR-treated sericin group exhibits significantly more new bone formation compared to the untreated sericin group [135].

Despite the promising results of this study, the findings cannot be directly applied to a clinical setting, as it was conducted on animals. However, animal studies can provide valuable predictive data for human clinical trials. The results of this study suggest potential clinical applications for 4HR-incorporated porcine bone graft materials, but more research and human trials are necessary to confirm their efficacy and safety. This research highlights the potential of 4HR-incorporated bone graft materials as a novel approach for bone regeneration and provides a foundation for further investigations in this area.

7.6 Closing Remark

The use of 4HR in tissue engineering holds considerable promise for improving biomaterial performance and promoting tissue regeneration outcomes. As a low-toxicity antiseptic agent, 4HR has shown potential in expediting the degradation of materials like silk fibroin, enhancing biodegradation of graft materials, and inhibiting foreign body reactions. Integrating 4HR into various biomaterials, such as silk fabric membranes, hydroxyapatite coatings, silk vascular patches, and silk sutures, has resulted in positive impacts on bone regeneration, infection resistance, reduced immune response, enhanced endothelium regeneration, and better knot-holding capacity with accelerated biodegradation.

Nonetheless, it is crucial to undertake more research to optimize 4HR concentration, application techniques, and the selection of biomaterials tailored for specific clinical settings. Long-term investigations are required to assess the full resorption of materials and gain a deeper understanding of 4HR's effects on tissue engineering applications. By expanding on existing knowledge and addressing the challenges, 4HR can become an integral element in the development of advanced biomaterials and tissue engineering approaches, ultimately improving patient outcomes and minimizing the necessity for additional surgical procedures.

References

1. Li Q, Lan P (2023) Activation of immune signals during organ transplantation. Signal Transduct Target Ther 8:110
2. Troeltzsch M, Troeltzsch M, Kauffmann P et al (2016) Clinical efficacy of grafting materials in alveolar ridge augmentation: a systematic review. J Craniomaxillofac Surg 44(10):1618–1629
3. Batoni E, Bonatti AF, De Maria C et al (2023) A computational model for the release of bioactive molecules by the hydrolytic degradation of a functionalized polyester-based scaffold. Pharmaceutics 15(3):815
4. Matsumoto A, Kajiya H, Yamamoto MN et al (2019) Degradation rate of DNA scaffolds and bone regeneration. J Biomed Mater Res B Appl Biomater 107(1):122–128
5. Wegner SV, Sentürk OI, Spatz JP (2015) Photocleavable linker for the patterning of bioactive molecules. Sci Rep 5:18309

6. Zhang H, Zhou L, Zhang W (2014) Control of scaffold degradation in tissue engineering: a review. Tissue Eng Part B Rev 20(5):492–502
7. Nikolaev YA, Tutel'yan AV, Loiko NG et al (2020) The use of 4-hexylresorcinol as antibiotic adjuvant. PLoS One 15(9):e0239147
8. Kim SG (2022) 4-hexylresorcinol: pharmacologic chaperone and its application for wound healing. Maxillofac Plast Reconstr Surg 44:5
9. Jo YY, Kweon H, Kim DW et al (2017) Accelerated biodegradation of silk sutures through matrix metalloproteinase activation by incorporating 4-hexylresorcinol. Sci Rep 7:42441
10. Jo YY, Kim DW, Choi JY, Kim SG (2019) 4-hexylresorcinol and silk sericin increase the expression of vascular endothelial growth factor via different pathways. Sci Rep 9:3448
11. Kazi S, Raptis S, Abbaspour F, Zeng W (2022) Foreign body-type giant cell reaction with extensive granulation tissue and intense inflammation after chemotherapy mimicking residual lymphoma on FDG PET. Eur J Hybrid Imaging 6:18
12. Eslami-Kaliji F, Hedayat Nia N, Lakey JR, Smink AM, Mohammadi M (2023) Mechanisms of foreign body giant cell formation in response to implantable biomaterials. Polymers 15:1313
13. Ahmadzadeh K, Vanoppen M, Rose C, Matthys P, Wouters C (2022) Multinucleated Giant cells: current insights in phenotype, biological activities, and mechanism of formation. Front Cell Dev Biol 10:724
14. Sheikh Z, Brooks PJ, Barzilay O, Fine N, Glogauer M (2015) Macrophages, foreign body giant cells and their response to implantable biomaterials. Materials 8:5671–5701
15. Jakubczyk K, Dec K, Kałduńska J, Kawczuga D, Kochman J, Janda K (2020) Reactive oxygen species—sources, functions, oxidative damage. Pol Merkur Lekarski 48:124–127
16. Ren X, Liu H, Wu X, Weng W, Wang X, Su J (2022) Reactive oxygen species (ROS)-responsive biomaterials for the treatment of bone-related diseases. Front Bioeng Biotechnol 9:820468
17. Shafiq M, Chen Y, Hashim R, He C, Mo X, Zhou X (2021) Reactive oxygen species-based biomaterials for regenerative medicine and tissue engineering applications. Front Bioeng Biotechnol 9:821288
18. Hasanuzzaman M, Raihan MRH, Masud AAC et al (2021) Regulation of reactive oxygen species and antioxidant defense in plants under salinity. Int J Mol Sci 22:9326
19. Hunyadi A (2019) The mechanism(s) of action of antioxidants: from scavenging reactive oxygen/nitrogen species to redox signaling and the generation of bioactive secondary metabolites. Med Res Rev 39:2505–2533
20. Liu Z, Ren Z, Zhang J et al (2018) Role of ROS and nutritional antioxidants in human diseases. Front Physiol 9:477
21. Zhi Z, Su Y, Xi Y et al (2017) Dual-functional polyethylene glycol-b-polyhexanide surface coating with in vitro and in vivo antimicrobial and antifouling activities. ACS Appl Mater Interfaces 9:10383–10397
22. McNally AK, Anderson JM (2003) Foreign body-type multinucleated giant cell formation is potently induced by alpha-tocopherol and prevented by the diacylglycerol kinase inhibitor R59022. Am J Pathol 163:1147–1156
23. Knight JA (2000) Review: free radicals, antioxidants, and the immune system. Ann Clin Lab Sci 30:145–158
24. Mrityunjaya M, Pavithra V, Neelam R, Janhavi P, Halami PM, Ravindra PV (2020) Immune-boosting, antioxidant and anti-inflammatory food supplements targeting pathogenesis of COVID-19. Front Immunol 11:570122
25. Brown J, Lu CL, Coburn J, Kaplan DL (2015) Impact of silk biomaterial structure on proteolysis. Acta Biomater 11:212–221
26. Kweon H, Kim SG, Choi JY (2014) Inhibition of foreign body giant cell formation by 4-hexylresorcinol through suppression of diacylglycerol kinase delta gene expression. Biomaterials 35:8576–8584
27. Sakai H, Sakane F (2012) Recent progress on type II diacylglycerol kinases: the physiological functions of diacylglycerol kinase delta, eta and kappa and their involvement in disease. J Biochem 152:397–406

28. Gassaway BM, Petersen MC, Surovtseva YV et al (2018) PKCε contributes to lipid-induced insulin resistance through cross talk with p70S6K and through previously unknown regulators of insulin signaling. Proc Natl Acad Sci USA 115:E8996–E9005
29. Carman GM, Kersting MC (2004) Phospholipid synthesis in yeast: regulation by phosphorylation. Biochem Cell Biol 82(1):62–70
30. Canton M, Sánchez-Rodríguez R, Spera I et al (2021) Reactive oxygen species in macrophages: sources and targets. Front Immunol 12:734229
31. Di Cera E (2009) Serine proteases. IUBMB Life 61(5):510–515
32. Vérollet C, Charrière GM, Labrousse A, Cougoule C, Le Cabec V, Maridonneau-Parini I (2011) Extracellular proteolysis in macrophage migration: losing grip for a breakthrough. Eur J Immunol 41(10):2805–2813
33. Skjøt-Arkil H, Barascuk N, Register T, Karsdal MA (2010) Macrophage-mediated proteolytic remodeling of the extracellular matrix in atherosclerosis results in neoepitopes: a potential new class of biochemical markers. Assay Drug Dev Technol 8(5):542–552
34. Kawano T, Inokuchi J, Eto M, Murata M, Kang JH (2021) Activators and inhibitors of protein kinase C (PKC): their applications in clinical trials. Pharmaceutics 13(11):1748
35. Mellor H, Parker P (1998) The extended protein kinase C superfamily. Biochem J 332:281
36. Zheleznyak A, Brown EJ (1992) Immunoglobulin-mediated phagocytosis by human monocytes requires protein kinase C activation. Evidence for protein kinase C translocation to phagosomes. J Biol Chem 267:12042
37. Larsen EC, DiGennaro JA, Saito N et al (2000) Differential requirement for classic and novel PKC isoforms in respiratory burst and phagocytosis in RAW 264.7 cells. J Immunol 165:2809
38. Lutz MA, Correll PH (2003) Activation of CR3-mediated phagocytosis by MSP requires the RON receptor, tyrosine kinase activity, phosphatidylinositol 3-kinase, and protein kinase C ζ. J Leukoc Biol 73:802
39. Kolczynska K, Loza-Valdes A, Hawro I, Sumara G (2020) Diacylglycerol-evoked activation of PKC and PKD isoforms in regulation of glucose and lipid metabolism: a review. Lipids Health Dis 19:113
40. Allen L, Aderem A (1996) Molecular definition of distinct cytoskeletal structures involved in complement- and fc receptor-mediated phagocytosis in macrophages. J Exp Med 184:627
41. Keranen LM, Dutil EM, Newton AC (1995) Protein kinase C is regulated in vivo by three functionally distinct phosphorylations. Curr Biol 5:1394
42. Tsutakawa SE, Medzihradszky KF, Flint AJ et al (1995) Determination of in vivo phosphorylation sites in protein kinase C. J Biol Chem 270:26807
43. Zhang F, Zhao G, Dong Z (2001) Phosphatidylcholine-specific phospholipase C and D in stimulation of RAW264.7 mouse macrophage like cells by lipopolysaccharide. Int Immunopharmacol 1(7):1375–1384
44. Aslam N, Alvi F (2019) How the DAG generation, transient shuttling of effector molecules and assembly of a signalosome at immunological synapse can regulate the early T cell response and L-selectin shedding? FASEB J 33(S1):802–807
45. McNally AK, Anderson JM (2011) Chapter 7. Macrophage fusion and multinucleated giant cells of inflammation. In: Dittmar T, Zänker KS (eds) Cell fusion in health and disease, advances in experimental medicine and biology, vol 713. Springer, Heidelberg, pp 97–111
46. Zachman AL, Page JM, Prabhakar G, Guelcher SA, Sung HJ (2013) Elucidation of adhesion-dependent spontaneous apoptosis in macrophages using phase separated PEG/polyurethane films. Acta Biomater 9(2):4964–4975
47. El Kebir D, Gjorstrup P, Filep JG (2012) Resolvin E1 promotes phagocytosis-induced neutrophil apoptosis and accelerates resolution of pulmonary inflammation. Proc Natl Acad Sci USA 109:14983–14988
48. Xiao W, Chen P, Wang R, Dong J (2013) Overload training inhibits phagocytosis and ROS generation of peritoneal macrophages: role of IGF-1 and MGF. Eur J Appl Physiol 113:117–125
49. Miura M, Hiwatashi N (1987) Impaired monocyte macrophages function in patients with Crohn's disease. J Clin Lab Immunol 24:167–170

50. Nakanishi-Matsui M, Yano S, Futai M (2013) Lipopolysaccharide-induced multinuclear cells: increased internalization of polystyrene beads and possible signals for cell fusion. Biochem Biophys Res Commun 440:611–616
51. Wang D, Xu Y, Li Q, Turng LS (2020) Artificial small-diameter blood vessels: materials, fabrication, surface modification, mechanical properties, and bioactive functionalities. J Mater Chem B 8:1801–1822
52. Sarkar S, Sales KM, Hamilton G, Seifalian AM (2007) Addressing thrombogenicity in vascular graft construction. J Biomed Mater Res B Appl Biomater 82:100–108
53. Kyriakides TR, Kim HJ, Zheng C, Harkins L, Tao W, Deschenes E (2022) Foreign body response to synthetic polymer biomaterials and the role of adaptive immunity. Biomed Mater 17:022007
54. Schwartz BS (1990) Heparin: what is it? How does it work? Clin Cardiol 13:VI12-VI15
55. Biran R, Pond D (2017) Heparin coatings for improving blood compatibility of medical devices. Adv Drug Deliv Rev 112:12–23
56. Gryglewski RJ (1995) Endothelial nitric oxide, prostacyclin (PGI2) and tissue plasminogen activator (t-PA): alliance or neutrality? Pol J Pharmacol 47:467–472
57. Maidoub H, Ben Mansour M, Chaubet F, Roudesli MS, Maaroufi RM (2009) Anticoagulant activity of a sulfated polysaccharide from the green alga arthrospira platensis. Biochim Biophys Acta 1790:1377–1381
58. Son MH, Park KH, Choi AR et al (2009) Investigation of biological activities of enzymatic hydrolysate of spirulina. J Korean Soc Food Sci Nutr 38:136–141
59. Park AR, Park YH, Kim HJ et al (2015) Tri-layered silk fibroin and poly-ε-caprolactone small diameter vascular grafts tested in vitro and in vivo. Macromol Res 23:924–936
60. Kweon H, Jo YY, Seok H et al (2017) In vivo bone regeneration ability of different layers of natural silk cocoon processed using an eco-friendly method. Macromol Res 25:806–816
61. Liu S, Dong C, Lu G et al (2013) Bilayered vascular grafts based on silk proteins. Acta Biomater 9:8991–9003
62. Chantawong P, Tanaka T, Uemura A et al (2017) Silk fibroin-pellethane® cardiovascular patches: effect of silk fibroin concentration on vascular remodeling in rat model. J Mater Sci Mater Med 28:191
63. Ha YY, Park YW, Kweon H, Jo YY, Kim SG (2014) Comparison of the physical properties and in vivo bioactivities of silkworm-cocoon-derived silk membrane, collagen membrane, and polytetrafluoroethylene membrane for guided bone regeneration. Macromol Res 22:1018–1023
64. Kim CW, Kim MK, Kim SG et al (2018) Angioplasty using 4-hexylresorcinol-incorporated silk vascular patch in rat carotid defect model. Appl Sci 8:2388
65. Cao Y, Wang B (2009) Biodegradation of silk biomaterials. Int J Mol Sci 10:1514–1524
66. Pérez-Rigueiro J, Elices M, Llorca J, Viney C (2001) Tensile properties of silkworm silk obtained by forced silking. J Appl Polym Sci 82:1928–1935
67. Lamboni L, Gauthier M, Yang G, Wang Q (2015) Silk sericin: a versatile material for tissue engineering and drug delivery. Biotechnol Adv 33:1855–1867
68. Bond R, Rerkasem K, Naylor AR, Aburahma AF, Rothwell PM (2004) Systematic review of randomized controlled trials of patch angioplasty versus primary closure and different types of patch materials during carotid endarterectomy. J Vasc Surg 40:1126–1135
69. Harrison GJ, How TV, Poole RJ et al (2014) Closure technique after carotid endarterectomy influences local hemodynamics. J Vasc Surg 60:418–427
70. Byrne J, Feustel P, Darling RC III (2007) In primary closure, routine patching, and eversion endarterectomy: what is the current state of the literature supporting use of these techniques? Semin Vasc Surg 20:226–235
71. Kang YJ, Noh JE, Lee MJ, Chae WS, Lee SY, Kim SG (2016) The effect of 4-hexylresorcinol on xenograft degradation in a rat calvarial defect model. Maxillofac Plast Reconstr Surg 38:29
72. Ahn J, Kim SG, Kim MK et al (2016) Topical delivery of 4-hexylresorcinol promotes wound healing via tumor necrosis factor-α suppression. Burns 42:1534–1541

73. Pye AD, Lockhart DE, Dawson MP, Murray CA, Smith AJ (2009) A review of dental implants and infection. J Hosp Infect 72:104–110
74. Bornstein MM, Cionca N, Mombelli A (2009) Systemic conditions and treatments as risks for implant therapy. Int J Oral Maxillofac Implants 24(Suppl):12–27
75. Yamashita D, Machigashira M, Miyamoto M et al (2009) Effect of surface roughness on initial responses of osteoblast-like cells on two types of zirconia. Dent Mater J 28:461–470
76. Hayes JS, Khan IM, Archer CW, Richards RG (2010) The role of surface microtopography in the modulation of osteoblast differentiation. Eur Cell Mater 20:98–108
77. Aykent F, Yondem I, Ozyesil AG, Gunal SK, Avunduk MC, Ozkan S (2010) Effect of different finishing techniques for restorative materials on surface roughness and bacterial adhesion. J Prosthet Dent 103:221–227
78. Burgers R, Gerlach T, Hahnel S, Schwarz F, Handel G, Gosau M (2010) In vivo and in vitro biofilm formation on two different titanium implant surfaces. Clin Oral Implants Res 21:156–164
79. Reynolds MA, Aichelmann-Reidy ME, Branch-Mays GL, Gunsolley JC (2003) The efficacy of bone replacement grafts in the treatment of periodontal osseous defects. A systematic review. Ann Periodontol 8:227–265
80. Jordan DR, Brownstein S, Faraji H (2004) Clinicopathologic analysis of 15 explanted hydroxyapatite implants. Ophthalmic Plast Reconstr Surg 20:285–290
81. Ganguli A, Steward C, Butler SL et al (2005) Bacterial adhesion to bisphosphonate-coated hydroxyapatite. J Mater Sci Mater Med 16:283–287
82. Fine DH, Furgang D, Kaplan J, Charlesworth J, Figurski DH (1999) Tenacious adhesion of Actinobacillus actinomycetemcomitans strain CU1000 to salivary-coated hydroxyapatite. Arch Oral Biol 44:1063–1076
83. Singh U, Grenier D, McBride BC (1989) Bacteroides gingivalis vesicles mediate attachment of Streptococci to serum-coated hydroxyapatite. Oral Microbiol Immunol 4:199–203
84. Thierer T, Davliakos JP, Keith JD Jr, Sanders JJ, Tarnow DP, Rivers JA (2008) Five-year prospective clinical evaluation of highly crystalline HA MP-1-coated dental implants. J Oral Implantol 34:39–46
85. Weyant RJ (2005) Multiple factors associated with HA-coated implants had more marginal bone loss but greater survival rates at 12 years than pure titanium implants. J Evid Based Dent Pract 5:198–199
86. Wheeler SL (1996) Eight-year clinical retrospective study of titanium plasma-sprayed and hydroxyapatite-coated cylinder implants. Int J Oral Maxillofac Implants 11:340–350
87. Lee EH, Ryu SM, Kim JY et al (2010) Effects of installation depth on survival of a hydroxyapatite-coated Bicon implant for single-tooth restoration. J Oral Maxillofac Surg 68:1345–1352
88. Evans RT, Baker PJ, Coburn RA, Fischman SL, Genco RJ (1977) In vitro antiplaque effects of antiseptic phenols. J Periodontol 48:156–162
89. Guandalini E, Ioppolo A, Mantovani A, Stacchini P, Giovannini C (1998) 4-hexylresorcinol as inhibitor of shrimp melanosis: efficacy and residues studies; evaluation of possible toxic effect in a human intestinal in vitro model (Caco-2); preliminary safety assessment. Food Addit Contam 15:171–180
90. Hahn BD, Lee JM, Park DS et al (2009) Mechanical and in vitro biological performances of hydroxyapatite-carbon nanotube composite coatings deposited on Ti by aerosol deposition. Acta Biomater 5:3205–3214
91. Kim SG, Hahn BD, Park DS et al (2011) Aerosol deposition of hydroxyapatite and 4-hexylresorcinol coatings on titanium alloys for dental implants. J Oral Maxillofac Surg 69:e354–e363
92. Leonard V (1925) The significance of hexylresorcinol and its homologues in relation to the problem of internal antisepsis. Science 62:408–412
93. Young CC, Damon SR (1927) Laboratory: the use of hexylresorcinol in the treatment of typhoid carriers. Am J Public Health 17:279–280

94. Hahn BD, Park DS, Choi JJ, Ryu J, Yoon WH, Lee BK (2009) Effect of the HA/β-TCP ratio on the biological performance of calcium phosphate ceramic coatings fabricated by a room-temperature powder spray in vacuum. J Am Ceram Soc 92:793–799
95. Som A, Yang L, Wong GC, Tew GN (2009) Divalent metal ion triggered activity of a synthetic antimicrobial in cardiolipin membranes. J Am Chem Soc 131:15102–15103
96. Kozubek A, Demel RA (1980) Permeability changes of erythrocytes and liposomes by 5-(n-alk(en)yl) resorcinols from rye. Biochim Biophys Acta 603:220–227
97. Muliukin AL, Sorokin VV, Loĭko NG et al (2002) Comparative study of the elemental composition of vegetative and resting microbial cells. Mikrobiologiia 71:37–48
98. Zemskov EA, Loukinova E, Mikhailenko I, Coleman RA, Strickland DK, Belkin AM (2009) Regulation of platelet-derived growth factor receptor function by integrin-associated cell surface transglutaminase. J Biol Chem 284:16693–16703
99. Yi W, Liu T, Gao X, Xie Y, Liu M (2021) 4-hexylresorcinol inhibits osteoclastogenesis by suppressing the NF-κB signaling pathway and reverses bone loss in ovariectomized mice. Exp Ther Med 21:354
100. Robinson HM Jr (1967) Effective antifungal drugs and indications for their use. Med Clin North Am 51:1181–1188
101. Moy RL, Waldman B, Hein DW (1992) A review of sutures and suturing techniques. J Dermatol Surg Oncol 18:785–795
102. Pillai CKS, Sharma CP (2010) Absorbable polymeric surgical sutures: chemistry, production, properties, biodegradability, and performances. J Biomater Appl 25:291–366
103. Dennis C, Sethu S, Nayak S, Mohan L, Morsi YY, Manivasagam G (2016) Suture materials-current and emerging trends. J Biomed Mater Res A 104:1544–1559
104. Chen X, Hou D, Tang X, Wang L (2015) Quantitative physical and handling characteristics of novel antibacterial braided silk suture materials. J Mech Behav Biomed Mater 50:160–170
105. Martínez-Alvarez O, Montero P, Gómez-Guillén C (2008) Evidence of an active laccase-like enzyme in deepwater pink shrimp (Parapenaeus longirostris). Food Chem 108:624–632
106. Kim DW, Jo YY, Garagiola U et al (2020) Increased level of vascular endothelial growth factors by 4-hexylresorcinol is mediated by transforming growth factor-β1 and accelerates capillary regeneration in the burns in diabetic animals. Int J Mol Sci 21(10):3473
107. Lee SW, Um IC, Kim SG, Cha MS (2015) Evaluation of bone formation and membrane degradation in guided bone regeneration using a 4-hexylresorcinol-incorporated silk fabric membrane. Maxillofac Plast Reconstr Surg 37:32
108. Amecke B, Bendix D, Entenmann G (1992) Resorbable polyesters: composition, properties, applications. Clin Mater 10:47–50
109. Okada T, Hayashi T, Ikada Y (1992) Degradation of collagen suture in vitro and in vivo. Biomaterials 13:448
110. Siasos G, Tousoulis D, Kioufis S et al (2012) Inflammatory mechanisms in atherosclerosis: the impact of matrix metalloproteinases. Curr Top Med Chem 12:1132–1148
111. Webster NL, Crowe SM (2006) Matrix metalloproteinases, their production by monocytes and macrophages and their potential role in HIV-related diseases. J Leukoc Biol 80:1052–1066
112. Durairaj RB (2005) Resorcinol: chemistry, technology and applications. Springer, Berlin, p 60
113. Krupianskiĭ YF, Yulmetov AR, Timofeev KN, Valeeva RA, Belova AV (2011) Effect of chemical chaperones on properties of lysozyme and the reaction center protein from Rhodobacter sphaeroides. Biofizika 56:13–30
114. Kim SG, Lee JH, Song KC et al (2011) 4-hexylresorcinol inhibits transglutaminase-2 activity and has synergistic effects along with cisplatin in KB cells. Oncol Rep 25:1597–1602
115. Kim SG, Song JY, Kweon H, Jo YY, Lee KG, Lee SW (2011) 4-hexylresorcinol inhibits NF-κB phosphorylation and has a synergistic effect with cisplatin in KB cells. Oncol Rep 26:1527–1532
116. Wang Y, Tang Z, Xue R et al (2011) TGF-β1 promoted MMP-2 mediated wound healing of anterior cruciate ligament fibroblasts through NF-κB. Connect Tissue Res 52:218–225
117. Hermann JS, Buser D (1996) Guided bone regeneration for dental implants. Curr Opin Periodontol 3:168–177

118. Lee SW, Kim SG (2014) Membranes for the guided bone regeneration. J Korean Assoc Maxillofac Plast Reconstr Surg 36:239–246
119. Song JY, Kim SG, Lee JW et al (2011) Accelerated healing with the use of a silk fibroin membrane for the guided bone regeneration technique. Oral Surg Oral Med Oral Pathol Oral Radiol Endod 112:e26–e33
120. Lee SW, Kim SG, Song JY et al (2013) Silk fibroin and 4-hexylresorcinol incorporation membrane for guided bone regeneration. J Craniofac Surg 24:1927–1930
121. McNally D, Shephard A, Field E (2012) Randomised, double-blind, placebo-controlled study of a single dose of an amylmetacresol/2, 4-dichlorobenzyl alcohol plus lidocaine lozenge or a hexylresorcinol lozenge for the treatment of acute sore throat due to upper respiratory tract infection. J Pharm Pharm Sci 15:281–294
122. Kundu B, Rajkhowa R, Kundu SC, Wang X (2013) Silk fibroin biomaterials for tissue regenerations. Adv Drug Deliv Rev 65:457–470
123. Altman GH, Diaz F, Jakuba C et al (2003) Silk-based biomaterials. Biomaterials 24:401–416
124. Aramwit P, Kanokpanont S, De-Eknamkul W, Srichana T (2009) Monitoring of inflammatory mediators induced by silk sericin. J Biosci Bioeng 107:556–561
125. Schwartzmann M (2000) Use of collagen membranes for guided bone regeneration: a review. Implant Dent 9:63–66
126. Postlethwait R (1970) Long-term comparative study of nonabsorbable sutures. Ann Surg 171:892–895
127. Lam K, Nijenhuis A, Bartels H et al (1995) Reinforced poly (L-lactic acid) fibres as suture material. J Appl Biomater 6:191–197
128. Salthouse TN, Matlaga BF, Wykoff MH (1977) Comparative tissue response to six suture materials in rabbit cornea, sclera, and ocular muscle. Am J Ophthalmol 84:224–233
129. Deodhar AK, Rana R (1997) Surgical physiology of wound healing: a review. J Postgrad Med 43:52–56
130. Dimitriou R, Mataliotakis GI, Angoules AG, Kanakaris NK, Giannoudis PV (2011) Complications following autologous bone graft harvesting from the iliac crest and using the RIA: a systematic review. Injury 42(Suppl 2):S3–S15
131. Kim MK, Park YT, Kim SG, Park YW, Lee SK, Choi WS (2012) The effect of a hydroxyapatite and 4-hexylresorcinol combination graft on bone regeneration in the rabbit calvarial defect model. J Kore Assoc Maxillofac Plast Reconstr Surg 34(6):377–383
132. Sohn HS, Oh JK (2019) Review of bone graft and bone substitutes with an emphasis on fracture surgeries. Biomater Res 23:9
133. Cooper GM, Kennedy MJ, Jamal B, Shields DW (2022) Autologous versus synthetic bone grafts for the surgical management of tibial plateau fractures: a systematic review and meta-analysis of randomized controlled trials. Bone Jt Open 3(3):218–228
134. Song JY, Kim SG, Park NR, Choi JY (2018) Porcine bone incorporated with 4-hexylresorcinol increases new bone formation by suppression of the nuclear factor kappa B signaling pathway. J Craniofac Surg 29:1983–1990
135. Lee JH, Kweon H, Oh JH et al (2022) 4-hexylresorcinol treatment before degumming increases the β-sheet structure of silk sericin and BMP-2 expression in RAW264.7 cells. Int J Mol Sci 24:150
136. Jo YY, Kweon H, Kim DW et al (2021) Silk sericin application increases bone morphogenic protein-2/4 expression via a toll-like receptor-mediated pathway. Int J Biol Macromol 190:607–617
137. Al-Halifa S, Zottig X, Babych M, Côté-Cyr M, Bourgault S, Archambault D (2020) Harnessing the activation of toll-like receptor 2/6 by self-assembled cross-β fibrils to design adjuvanted nanovaccines. Nano 10:1981
138. Kang YJ, Yang WG, Chae WS, Kim DW, Kim SG, Rotaru H (2022) Administration of 4-hexylresorcinol increases p53-mediated transcriptional activity in oral cancer cells with the p53 mutation. Oncol Rep 48:160

Chapter 8
The Application of 4-Hexylresorcinol for Preventing Diabetic Complications

Abstract This chapter explores the effects of 4-hexylresorcinol (4HR) on various diabetes-related complications in animal models. Diabetes can negatively impact multiple organ systems, including the liver, male reproductive system, kidneys, and bones. The study investigates the potential benefits of 4HR administration in mitigating these complications. Findings suggest that 4HR may help alleviate liver damage and mitigate male reproductive system issues in diabetic animals. Additionally, 4HR appears to have a positive effect on diabetic nephropathy, possibly by reducing oxidative stress and inflammation. In terms of bone complications, 4HR administration has been associated with increased cortical bone thickness in diabetic animals, possibly through anti-inflammatory, antioxidant, or bone remodeling effects. Overall, this study highlights the potential therapeutic benefits of 4HR in managing diabetes-related complications. However, further research is needed to confirm the exact mechanisms and optimize the use of 4HR in clinical settings.

Keywords 4-Hexylresorcinol (4HR) · Diabetes-related complications · Male reproductive system · Diabetic nephropathy · Oxidative stress

Mitochondria contain their own unique DNA and can replicate within a cell's cytoplasm [1]. Present exclusively in eukaryotic cells and absent in prokaryotic cells, mitochondria are considered a form of symbiosis within eukaryotic cells [2]. As the primary cellular powerhouse, they produce adenosine triphosphate (ATP) from glucose, fueling the cell's energy requirements [1]. When administered as a microbial dormancy inducer, 4-hexylresorcinol (4HR) can impact mitochondrial function [3]. Upon 4HR administration, it is expected to inhibit mitochondrial respiration, subsequently reducing the production of reactive oxygen species (ROS), which are by-products of mitochondrial respiration [4].

Mitochondrial function can be altered in diabetes mellitus (DM). Mitochondria are the primary cellular organelles responsible for generating energy in the form of ATP through oxidative phosphorylation [1]. Glucose metabolism, particularly in the form of glycolysis and the tricarboxylic acid (TCA) cycle, provides the substrates needed for oxidative phosphorylation in the mitochondria [5]. In both type 1 and

S.-G. Kim, *Biomedical Application of 4-Hexylresorcinol*,
https://doi.org/10.1007/978-981-97-0637-2_8

type 2 diabetes, changes in mitochondrial function have been observed and are thought to contribute to the development and progression of the disease and its complications:

1. Impaired mitochondrial bioenergetics: Impaired mitochondrial bioenergetics is a significant factor in the development and progression of diabetes. Elevated blood sugar levels and impaired insulin signaling in diabetes disrupt the normal metabolic processes within mitochondria, leading to reduced ATP production efficiency [6]. This compromised bioenergetics results in decreased cellular energy availability, which has profound implications for cellular function and overall metabolic homeostasis in individuals with diabetes. A consequence of impaired mitochondrial bioenergetics in diabetes is the increased production of ROS. These highly reactive molecules can cause extensive damage to cellular components such as proteins, lipids, and DNA [7]. The overproduction of ROS, coupled with a decline in antioxidant capacity, contributes to oxidative stress, a hallmark of diabetic complications. The consequences of impaired mitochondrial bioenergetics extend beyond cellular damage. Decreased ATP production can affect various tissues and organs, leading to systemic metabolic dysfunction. For instance, reduced availability of ATP can hinder cellular glucose uptake, leading to elevated blood sugar levels and contributing to the development of insulin resistance. Moreover, the impaired mitochondrial metabolism in diabetes can also impact lipid metabolism, resulting in lipid disturbances and abnormalities in lipid storage and utilization.
2. Mitochondrial oxidative stress: Mitochondrial oxidative stress is a recognized consequence of high blood sugar levels and dysfunctional mitochondria, leading to an increase in ROS production. This elevation in ROS overwhelms the cell's antioxidant defense mechanisms, resulting in oxidative stress [8]. Oxidative stress, in turn, has been implicated in the pathogenesis of insulin resistance, pancreatic beta-cell dysfunction, and the development of various diabetic complications such as nephropathy, retinopathy, neuropathy, and cardiovascular disease [9, 10]. The accumulation of ROS within the mitochondria occurs due to impaired electron transport chain function, resulting in leakage of electrons and subsequent ROS generation. ROS, including superoxide anion and hydrogen peroxide, can damage mitochondrial proteins, lipids, and nucleic acids, leading to mitochondrial dysfunction. Furthermore, mitochondrial DNA mutations, which are more susceptible to oxidative damage due to their proximity to ROS-producing sites, can further exacerbate mitochondrial dysfunction and ROS generation, perpetuating a cycle of oxidative stress and cellular damage. This sustained oxidative stress can have deleterious effects on insulin signaling pathways, impairing glucose uptake and utilization. Additionally, pancreatic beta-cell function can be compromised by oxidative stress, resulting in reduced insulin secretion, and further exacerbating hyperglycemia. Furthermore, oxidative stress-induced damage to renal, retinal, neuropathic, and cardiovascular tissues contributes to the development of diabetic complications.

3. Mitochondrial dynamics and morphology: Diabetes mellitus is a complex metabolic disorder that is characterized by elevated blood glucose levels due to impaired insulin secretion or insulin resistance. In recent years, there has been growing evidence suggesting a crucial link between diabetes and mitochondrial dysfunction. Specifically, diabetes can disrupt the delicate balance between mitochondrial fusion and fission, resulting in changes in mitochondrial morphology and impaired mitochondrial function [11]. Mitochondrial dynamics, which encompass the processes of fusion (joining of mitochondria) and fission (division of mitochondria), play a fundamental role in maintaining mitochondrial health and function. Disruption of these processes can have detrimental effects on cellular metabolism, including impaired glucose uptake and utilization. Research has shown that in diabetic individuals, there is a shift toward increased mitochondrial fission and reduced fusion, leading to fragmented and dysfunctional mitochondria [11]. Impaired mitochondrial dynamics have been associated with insulin resistance, a key feature of type 2 diabetes. Insulin resistance occurs when the body's cells become less responsive to the actions of insulin, resulting in reduced glucose uptake and utilization. Studies have shown that dysfunctional mitochondria, characterized by abnormal morphology and impaired function, contribute to insulin resistance by disrupting cellular energy metabolism and impairing insulin signaling pathways. Furthermore, alterations in mitochondrial dynamics have also been implicated in the development of diabetic complications [12]. Mitochondrial dysfunction has been associated with oxidative stress, inflammation, and endothelial dysfunction, which are all key factors contributing to the pathogenesis of diabetic complications, such as nephropathy, retinopathy, and neuropathy.
4. Mitochondrial biogenesis: Diabetes, a chronic metabolic disorder, has been shown to have a detrimental impact on mitochondrial biogenesis, the process responsible for the formation of new mitochondria [13]. This impairment in mitochondrial biogenesis can have significant consequences on the overall functioning of mitochondria in cells. Research suggests that reduced mitochondrial biogenesis in diabetes contributes to the development of mitochondrial dysfunction, decreased energy production, and increased oxidative stress. Mitochondria are crucial organelles responsible for generating energy in the form of ATP through oxidative phosphorylation. Impaired mitochondrial biogenesis leads to fewer mitochondria, resulting in diminished capacity for ATP synthesis. This directly affects cellular energy production, leading to a lack of energy supply for various cellular processes. Consequently, individuals with diabetes may experience fatigue, muscle weakness, and a reduction in physical endurance. Furthermore, reduced mitochondrial biogenesis in diabetes has been associated with mitochondrial dysfunction. Mitochondrial dysfunction manifests as an impaired ability of mitochondria to effectively carry out their metabolic functions. This can result in an imbalance between ROS production and antioxidant defenses within the mitochondria, leading to increased oxidative stress. Oxidative

stress, characterized by an excess of ROS, can damage cellular structures, including proteins, lipids, and DNA, and ultimately contribute to the development and progression of complications associated with diabetes, such as cardiovascular disease and neuropathy [14].

Targeting mitochondrial function has been proposed as a potential therapeutic strategy for the prevention and treatment of diabetes and its complications [14, 15]. Approaches under investigation include enhancing mitochondrial bioenergetics, reducing oxidative stress, and promoting mitochondrial biogenesis. However, more research is needed to develop effective mitochondrial-targeted therapies and to fully understand their potential impact on diabetes management.

When a drug stimulates glycolysis while inhibiting mitochondrial respiration, it may not result in a significant decrease in ATP production. The activation of glycolysis can compensate for the diminished ATP generation caused by the suppression of mitochondrial respiration. Simultaneously, reducing mitochondrial ROS production could be advantageous in limiting the oxidative stress related to diabetes. By decreasing mitochondrial ROS production, it may be possible to protect cellular components like proteins, lipids, and DNA from oxidative damage, potentially mitigating diabetes-associated complications such as nephropathy, retinopathy, neuropathy, and cardiovascular disease.

This approach, although promising in reducing mitochondrial ROS production for potential benefits in diabetes treatment, raises concerns regarding the potential downsides associated with decreased ATP production and inhibition of the TCA cycle. ATP is pivotal in cellular energy metabolism and acts as a fuel for various cellular processes. Any disruption in the generation of ATP can negatively impact cell function and overall health. A reduction in ATP production can lead to a decline in cellular energy availability, which can hinder essential cellular processes such as protein synthesis, DNA replication, and maintenance of membrane potential. These processes are crucial for normal cellular function, and any impairment in them can have detrimental effects on overall cellular and organismal health. Additionally, the inhibition of the TCA cycle can further exacerbate the decrease in ATP production as it is the primary generator of reducing equivalents, which are necessary for ATP synthesis through oxidative phosphorylation. Moreover, diminished ATP production and TCA cycle inhibition may have far-reaching consequences beyond energy metabolism. ATP is an essential cofactor in numerous enzymatic reactions and signaling pathways. A decrease in ATP levels can disrupt the functionality of ATP-dependent enzymes and affect cellular signaling processes, potentially leading to further complications in cellular function and overall health.

To fully assess the potential risks associated with reduced ATP production and TCA cycle inhibition, rigorous evaluation is necessary. This evaluation should consider the balance between the benefits of decreased ROS production and the potential detrimental effects on cellular energy metabolism and overall health. Additionally, the identification of alternative strategies that can mitigate the downsides of this approach while still targeting mitochondrial ROS production could provide a more comprehensive perspective in diabetes treatment.

The therapeutic effects of 4HR on diabetes mellitus were first reported in a 2022 publication [16]. This paper primarily aimed to investigate the anti-leukemia effects of 4HR [16]. Due to 4HR's inhibitory action on α-glycosidase and sorbitol dehydrogenase observed in the study, the authors suggested that 4HR might possess antidiabetic properties [16]. Prior to this publication, a 2020 patent had already claimed the therapeutic effects of 4HR on diabetes [17]. According to the patent, the primary mechanism underlying 4HR's antidiabetic properties involves sirtuin (SIRT) activation and the inhibition of class I and II histone deacetylases [17].

During a seminar at Kyungpook National University on December 20, 2021, Prof. Je-Yong Choi shared intriguing research findings. Prof. Choi aimed to identify potential target proteins for 4HR. In his search, he discovered that among the tested proteins, glyceraldehyde 3-phosphate dehydrogenase (GAPDH) exhibited strongest affinity for 4HR among screened proteins. Subsequent enzyme activity analyses revealed that 4HR acts as a potent activator of GAPDH, rather than an inhibitor. GAPDH is a key enzyme for glycolysis [18]. As a result, 4HR administration can enhance glycolysis and ATP production, even when mitochondrial function is inhibited (Fig. 8.1).

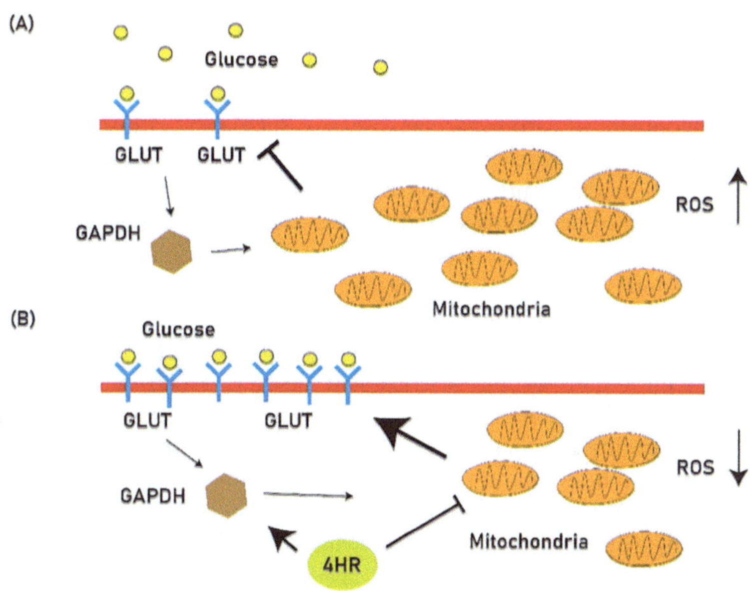

Fig. 8.1 Suggested mechanism for metabolic restriction mediated by 4HR: (**a**) In conditions abundant with nutrients, there is an excess of glucose in the bloodstream. If all of it is taken up by cells, mitochondria will be overloaded, leading to increased production of reactive oxygen species (ROS). To prevent excessive glucose entry, the expression level of glucose transporter proteins (GLUT) is decreased. Consequently, high blood sugar levels are maintained. (**b**) When 4HR is administered to cells, mitochondrial respiration and subsequent ROS production are inhibited. Moreover, 4HR could enhance GLUT expression through the suppression of histone deacetylase, thereby promoting the extraction of additional glucose from the bloodstream. The imported glucose is metabolized by GAPDH, which is activated by 4HR

In addition, the inhibition of mitochondrial function by 4HR can indirectly influence the expression of glucose transporters (GLUTs). Mitochondrial dysfunction and the resulting energy deficit in the cell can activate AMP-activated protein kinase (AMPK), a cellular energy sensor [19]. When activated, AMPK initiates a cascade of events to restore energy balance. One of the consequences of AMPK activation is the increased translocation and expression of GLUT4, the major glucose transporter in muscle and adipose tissue [20]. Additionally, 4HR may boost GLUT4 expression in liver by inhibiting histone deacetylase, thus facilitating the removal of extra glucose from the bloodstream. This response could lead to improved glucose uptake and utilization in these tissues, potentially providing some benefits in diabetes management such as decreasing blood sugar level. Consequently, plans were made to conduct experiments using a diabetic animal model.

8.1 Diabetes-Associated Complications

Diabetes is a chronic condition that can lead to various complications if not managed properly. These complications can affect different parts of the body and impact overall health. Some common complications associated with diabetes include:

1. Cardiovascular disease: One of the most significant risks posed by diabetes is the development of cardiovascular diseases, such as heart disease, stroke, and peripheral artery disease (PAD). As outlined in various studies, diabetes plays a crucial role in damaging blood vessels and impairing blood flow, thereby increasing the susceptibility of individuals to these life-threatening conditions [21]. The detrimental effects of diabetes on blood vessels can be attributed to several underlying mechanisms. Chronic high blood sugar levels, a characteristic feature of diabetes, contribute to the accumulation of fatty deposits in the artery walls, a condition known as atherosclerosis. Over time, the buildup of these plaques narrows the arteries and restricts blood flow. Additionally, diabetes-related inflammation and oxidative stress further exacerbate vascular damage, leading to endothelial dysfunction and impaired vasodilation. Consequently, the compromised blood flow predisposes individuals with diabetes to an increased risk of heart disease, stroke, and PAD [21].
2. Neuropathy: High blood sugar levels, a characteristic feature of diabetes, have been known to have detrimental effects on nerve function, particularly in the lower extremities such as the legs and feet [22, 23]. This condition, known as diabetic neuropathy, is a major complication of diabetes that can have serious consequences. One of the most significant consequences of diabetic neuropathy is the development of pain and numbness in the affected areas. Patients may experience a burning or tingling sensation, or even complete loss of sensation, making it difficult for them to detect injuries or changes in temperature. This can lead to delayed wound healing and an increased risk of developing ulcers or infections [22].
3. Kidney damage (nephropathy): Diabetes has been identified as a significant risk factor for the development of kidney disease [24]. The kidneys play a crucial

role in maintaining the body's fluid balance and filtering waste products from the blood. However, in people with diabetes, the prolonged exposure to high levels of blood sugar can cause damage to the small blood vessels and capillaries in the kidneys. This damage can impair the kidneys' filtration system, leading to the development of kidney disease. In the early stages, diabetes-related kidney disease may not cause any noticeable symptoms. However, as the condition progresses, symptoms such as increased urination, fatigue, swelling in the legs and feet, and high blood pressure may occur. It is essential for individuals with diabetes to regularly monitor their kidney function through routine urine and blood tests to detect kidney damage at an early stage. Early detection is crucial, as it allows for prompt interventions to slow down the progression of kidney disease. In severe cases, diabetes-related kidney disease can lead to kidney failure, which requires either dialysis or kidney transplantation for survival. This condition, known as end-stage renal disease (ESRD), significantly impacts an individual's quality of life and places a significant burden on healthcare systems. Therefore, preventing or delaying the onset of kidney disease in individuals with diabetes is of utmost importance [24]. This can be achieved through effective management of blood sugar levels, blood pressure control, and regular medical check-ups.

4. Retinopathy: High blood sugar can damage the blood vessels in the retina, leading to vision problems or even blindness [25].
5. Foot problems: Poor blood flow and nerve damage in the feet can lead to ulcers, infections, and deformities, which can be challenging to treat and may require amputation in extreme cases [26].
6. Skin conditions: Diabetes can cause skin problems like bacterial and fungal infections, as well as affect the skin's ability to heal properly [27].
7. Hearing impairment: Diabetes may increase the risk of hearing problems due to nerve damage and poor blood flow to the inner ear [28].
8. Sleep apnea: Diabetes can contribute to the development of obstructive sleep apnea, a condition in which breathing repeatedly stops and starts during sleep [29].
9. Depression: The emotional and physical toll of managing diabetes can lead to an increased risk of depression [30].
10. Gastroparesis: Gastroparesis refers to delayed gastric emptying, a condition where the stomach takes longer than normal to move food into the small intestine. This can occur when the nerves that regulate stomach muscle contractions are damaged by the elevated blood sugar levels often seen in diabetes. As a result, the stomach's ability to efficiently empty its contents is compromised. This impairment in gastric motility can cause a range of symptoms, such as nausea, vomiting, bloating, and early satiety. The presence of gastroparesis in individuals with diabetes can further complicate glycemic control [31]. Delayed stomach emptying can lead to inconsistent or erratic absorption of ingested carbohydrates, making it challenging to predict and manage blood sugar levels effectively. Moreover, the delayed delivery of food from the stomach to the

intestines can contribute to postprandial hyperglycemia, leading to spikes in blood sugar that are difficult to control. These fluctuations in blood glucose levels can exacerbate symptoms, making it even more challenging for individuals with diabetes to maintain adequate glycemic control.

11. Taste disorder: DM has been shown to affect taste perceptions by altering taste thresholds for various taste modalities. Studies have reported changes in taste thresholds for substances like hydrochloric acid, sucrose, sodium chloride, and urea in diabetic subjects [32, 33]. Sensory impairments, including taste disorders, are commonly observed complications in DM. These deficits occur early in the disease course and are generalized, affecting both tactile and special senses like taste.

In addition to abovementioned complications, the bone, salivary gland, and testis are influenced by DM.

8.2 The Control of Blood Sugar Level by 4HR

In individuals with diabetes, elevated blood sugar levels arise from issues related to insulin, a hormone generated by the pancreas that aids in regulating blood sugar. When insulin interacts with its receptor, the glucose transporter protein GLUT relocates to the cell membrane [34]. As GLUT facilitates glucose transport, cells absorb glucose from the bloodstream to use as energy or store it for future needs. There are two main types of diabetes that lead to elevated blood sugar levels: type 1 diabetes and type 2 diabetes.

In type 1 diabetes, the body's immune system mistakenly attacks and destroys the insulin-producing beta cells in the pancreas [35]. As a result, little or no insulin is produced. Without insulin, cells cannot take in glucose from the bloodstream, causing blood sugar levels to rise. People with type 1 diabetes must take insulin injections or use an insulin pump to replace the missing insulin and maintain blood sugar levels within a target range.

Type 2 diabetes is linked to an excess of nutrients [36]. When individuals consume more food than their body requires, an excess of glucose is present in the bloodstream. This glucose can enter cells, but mitochondrial overload can lead to the suppression of GLUT expression [37]. As a result, cells become less responsive to insulin signals, a condition known as insulin resistance. In the initial stages of type 2 diabetes, the pancreas compensates for the diminished effectiveness of insulin by producing more of it [38]. However, over time, the pancreas may struggle to meet the increased demand for insulin, resulting in a relative insulin deficiency. Both insulin resistance and inadequate insulin production contribute to the elevated blood sugar levels observed in people with type 2 diabetes.

In the diabetic model, a total of 40 rats (7 weeks old) were utilized for the study, comprising 20 males and 20 females. The study was approved by the GWNU IACUC (approval #: GWNU-2021-22, approval date: November 23, 2021). Diabetes was induced in all animals via intravenous injection of streptozotocin (STZ: 40 mg/kg). Three days after STZ injection, fasting serum glucose levels were measured. Animals with serum glucose levels >300 mg/dl met the inclusion criteria and were randomly assigned to control or experimental groups. The experimental group received 5 mg/kg of 4HR through subcutaneous injection twice weekly, while the control group received a corresponding volume of 4HR solvent. On designated study days and following overnight fasting, tail vein blood samples were collected, and fasting blood glucose (FBG) levels were determined using a digital glucometer. Animals exhibiting weight loss greater than 20% compared to the previous measurement were considered deceased; otherwise, the experiment proceeded for 12 weeks. As many rats in the control group showed serious weight loss, animal experiments were stopped at 9 weeks after STZ injection.

Before euthanizing the animals, a glucose tolerance test was conducted. After obtaining FBG measurements, a 2 g/kg dose of glucose solution was orally administered to the rats on the final study day. Blood glucose levels were then assessed at 60- and 120-minutes post-glucose consumption. A digital glucometer (GLUCOCARD, ARKRAY, Japan) was used to measure glucose levels, and the area under the glycemic curve (AUC) index was calculated to represent the overall increase in glucose concentrations following glucose ingestion. Blood samples were collected, immediately centrifuged, and the serum + lysis buffer (1:1, vol to vol) mixture was stored for subsequent analysis. Blinding techniques were employed during data collection and analysis.

For comparative purposes, non-diabetic groups were included. In a separate study approved by the GWNU IACUC (approval #: GWNU-2021-21, approval date: November 23, 2021), a total of 20 male rats (4 weeks old) were used. These animals did not receive STZ injections. The experimental group received 5 mg/kg of 4HR via subcutaneous injection twice a week, while the control group received an equivalent volume of 4HR solvent. The same euthanasia criteria applied to the diabetic study were followed.

At the time of euthanasia, the age of animal in both DM and heathy groups was 16 weeks old. After euthanizing the animals, tissue samples were collected from the liver, kidney, pancreas, testis, femur, eyeball, and head for further examination. One portion of the collected tissue was immersed in formalin for fixation, while another portion was stored in a deep freezer for subsequent Western blot analysis.

In both forms of diabetes, it is crucial to manage blood sugar levels through a combination of medication, diet, and exercise to prevent complications and maintain overall health. In our animal experiment, female rats recovered from the diabetic condition, leading to the inclusion of only male rats for further study. No significant differences were observed between the groups in fasting and 1-h post-loading blood sugar levels ($P > 0.05$). However, the 4HR-treated group demonstrated a blood sugar level of 710.8 ± 110.8 mg/dL, while the untreated control group displayed 954.7 ± 76.9 mg/dL (Fig. 8.2). This difference between the groups was statistically significant ($P = 0.001$).

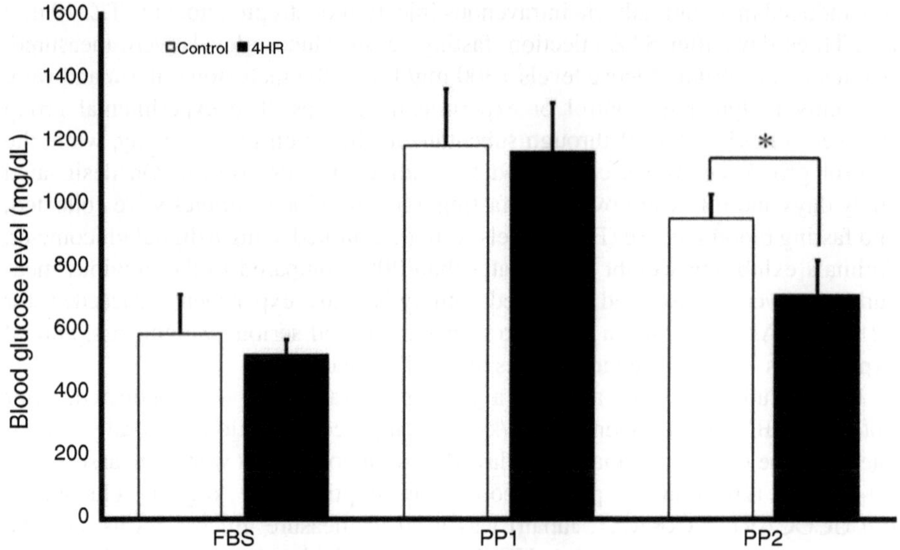

Fig. 8.2 Blood sugar levels in diabetic male rats. No significant differences were observed between groups in fasting blood sugar (FBS) levels. Following glucose administration, both groups exhibited increased blood sugar levels at 1-h post-loading (PP1). Notably, a significant difference was detected at 2 h post-loading (PP2), with the 4HR-treated group showing significantly lower values compared to the untreated control group (*$P < 0.05$)

Weight loss can indeed be observed in individuals with diabetes, particularly when the condition is undiagnosed or poorly managed. This phenomenon can be attributed to several factors. In both types of diabetes, the inability of glucose to effectively enter cells prompts the body to break down fat and muscle tissue for energy, leading to weight loss [39]. Elevated blood sugar levels can result in increased urine production as the body endeavours to eliminate surplus glucose [40]. Consequently, calories and fluids are lost, contributing to weight loss.

Body weight changes were monitored weekly (Fig. 8.3). In healthy animals, 4HR treatment led to a slower rate of weight gain compared to the untreated control group, which is consistent with our previous publication [41]. In contrast, this trend was reversed in the DM animal model. The administration of 4HR appeared to attenuate DM-induced weight loss. The 4HR group experienced a smaller weight loss compared to the untreated control group in the context of DM (Fig. 8.3).

GLUT plays a crucial role in the uptake of glucose by cells. These proteins are responsible for transporting glucose across the cell membrane, allowing glucose to enter the cell, and be used for energy or stored for later use [42]. There are several types of GLUT proteins, each with specific tissue distribution and functions. The two most well-known GLUT proteins, GLUT1 and GLUT4, have distinct roles in glucose transport.

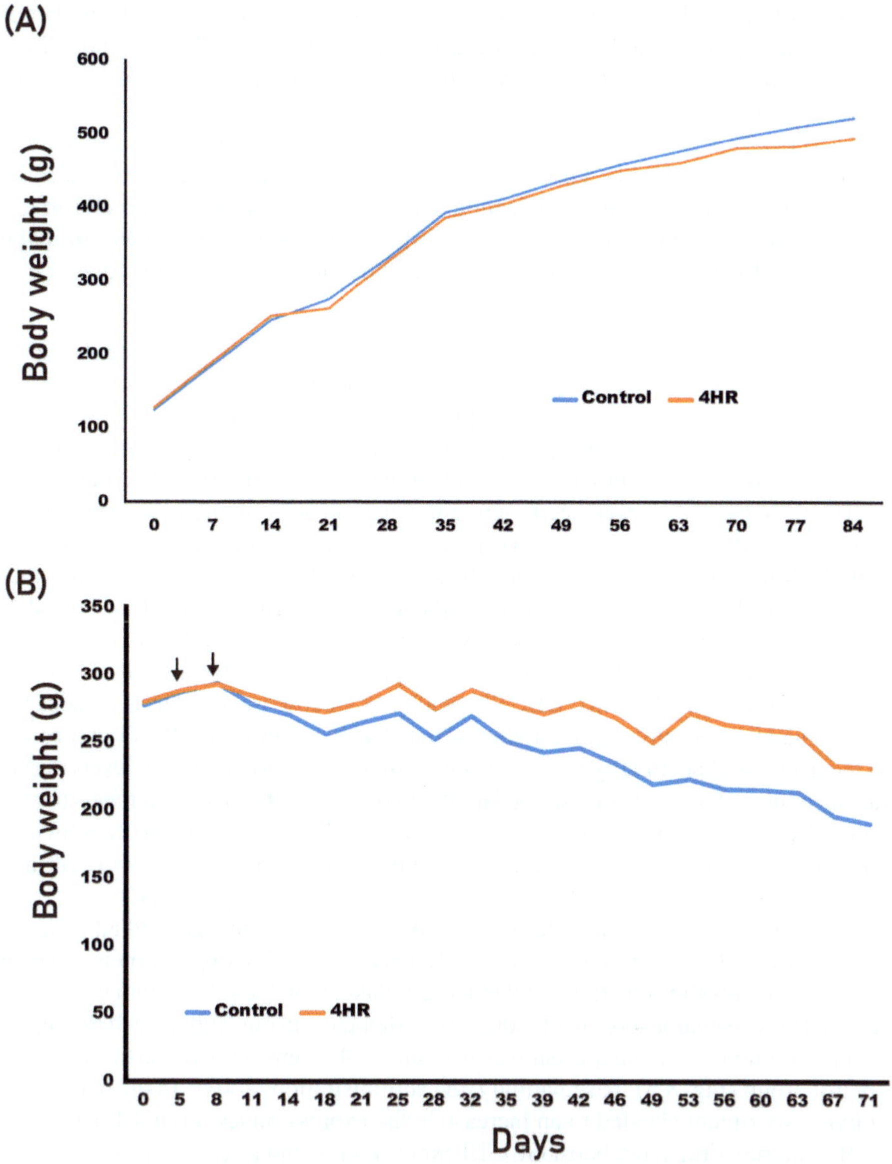

Fig. 8.3 Alterations in body weight. (**a**) In healthy animals, body weight steadily increased with age. The average body weight in the 4HR group was slightly lower than that of the untreated control group. (**b**) In the case of DM animals, body weight did not increase; instead, it consistently decreased with age. Compared to the untreated control group, the 4HR group experienced less weight loss due to DM. Arrows denote the time points of STZ injections

1. GLUT1: This glucose transporter is widely distributed throughout the body and is primarily responsible for basal glucose uptake in most cells [42]. GLUT1 is especially important for the brain, as it facilitates the transport of glucose across the blood-brain barrier [42, 43].
2. GLUT4: This glucose transporter is primarily found in the muscle and adipose (fat) tissue [44]. Unlike GLUT1, the activity of GLUT4 is highly regulated by insulin [45]. In the presence of insulin, GLUT4 is translocated to the cell surface, allowing glucose to enter the cell [44, 45]. This mechanism is critical for maintaining blood sugar levels after a meal, as it enables the efficient uptake of glucose by muscle and fat cells.

In the context of diabetes, the role of GLUT4 is particularly important. In type 2 diabetes, insulin resistance impairs the ability of GLUT4 to translocate to the cell surface, leading to decreased glucose uptake by muscle and fat cells and resulting in elevated blood sugar levels [46]. Improving insulin sensitivity can enhance GLUT4 function and help lower blood sugar levels in individuals with type 2 diabetes.

The liver plays a central role in glucose metabolism. It maintains blood glucose levels by balancing gluconeogenesis (the production of glucose from non-carbohydrate sources) and glycogenolysis (the breakdown of glycogen into glucose) during fasting, and glycogenesis (the storage of glucose as glycogen) after meals [46]. The liver is also a site of insulin clearance and degradation.

In the context of diabetes, enhancing the expression of GLUT1 and GLUT4 in the liver may offer some benefits. GLUT1, as a basal glucose transporter, is responsible for maintaining a steady supply of glucose to cells [44]. Elevating GLUT1 expression in the liver could potentially assist in better regulation of blood glucose levels during fasting or periods of low glucose availability. In our study, the diabetic animals treated with 4HR exhibited an increased expression level of GLUT1 compared to the untreated control group (Fig. 8.4). Nonetheless, the administration of 4HR did not result in a higher expression level of GLUT1 in the hepatocyte culture experiment.

Even though GLUT4 is predominantly expressed in the muscle and adipose tissue, it can also be found in the liver [47]. Enhancing GLUT4 expression in the liver may enhance insulin sensitivity and glucose uptake, which could potentially lead to reduced blood sugar levels in individuals with diabetes. In our study, the 4HR-treated group exhibited a higher expression level of GLUT4 when compared to the untreated control group (Fig. 8.5). Fascinatingly, the administration of 4HR in the hepatocyte culture experiment also led to an increase in the expression level of GLUT4.

By utilizing drugs that boost GLUT4 expression or enhance its translocation and activity, it may be possible to augment glucose uptake and reduce blood sugar levels. In fact, some medications currently used for type 2 diabetes are believed to function, at least partially, by improving GLUT4 performance. Thiazolidinediones (TZDs), for example, serve as insulin sensitizers by activating a nuclear receptor called peroxisome proliferator-activated receptor gamma (PPAR-γ) [48]. PPAR-γ activation results in elevated GLUT4 expression and enhanced insulin sensitivity, which in turn promotes glucose uptake by muscle and fat cells [49]. As 4HR increased the expression level of GLUT1 and 4 in the liver, this will be helpful for reducing blood sugar level.

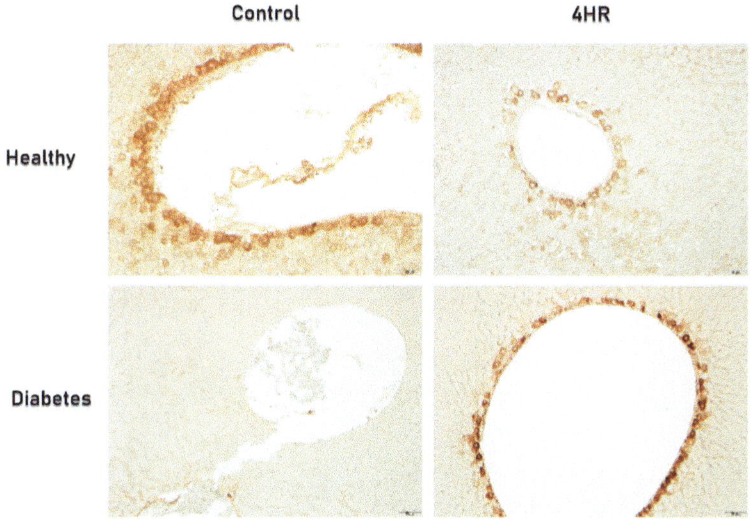

Fig. 8.4 Expression levels of GLUT1 in the liver. In healthy animals, both groups exhibited GLUT1 expression surrounding the portal system. In diabetic animals, the untreated control group displayed lower GLUT1 expression levels compared to the 4HR group (original magnification ×200)

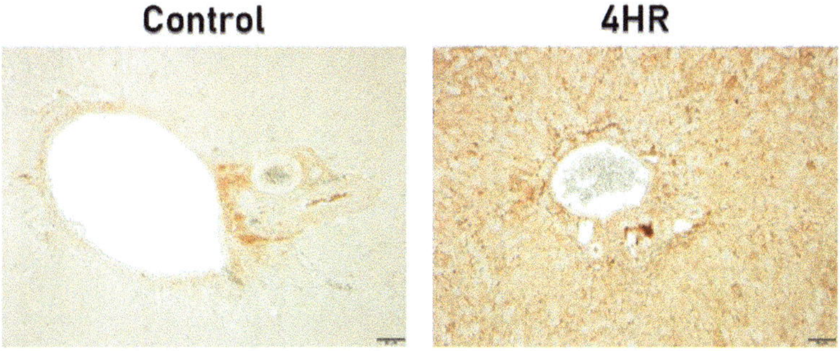

Fig. 8.5 Expression levels of GLUT4 in the liver of diabetic animal model. The untreated control group displayed lower GLUT1 expression levels compared to the 4HR group (original magnification ×200)

The results of the immunoprecipitation-high-performance liquid chromatography (IP-HPLC) analysis using blood serum are presented in Fig. 8.6. In normal rats, 4HR increased insulin levels by 23.3%, energy expenditure proteins (GAPDH by 6.3% and LGR4 by 11.3%), antiaging and protective proteins (FOXO3 by 23.3%, sirtuin 1 by 23.2%, and klotho by 8.7%), and the anti-obesity protein leptin by 5.8%. Meanwhile, it decreased the first-step glucose metabolism enzyme HKII by 3.3% (Fig. 8.6a, b). In terms of 4HR's effect on DM-induced rats, it upregulated HKII by 27.8%, sirtuin 1 by 13.4%, FOXO3 by 15.4%, and klotho by 5.9% in DM-induced female rats (Fig. 8.6c, d).

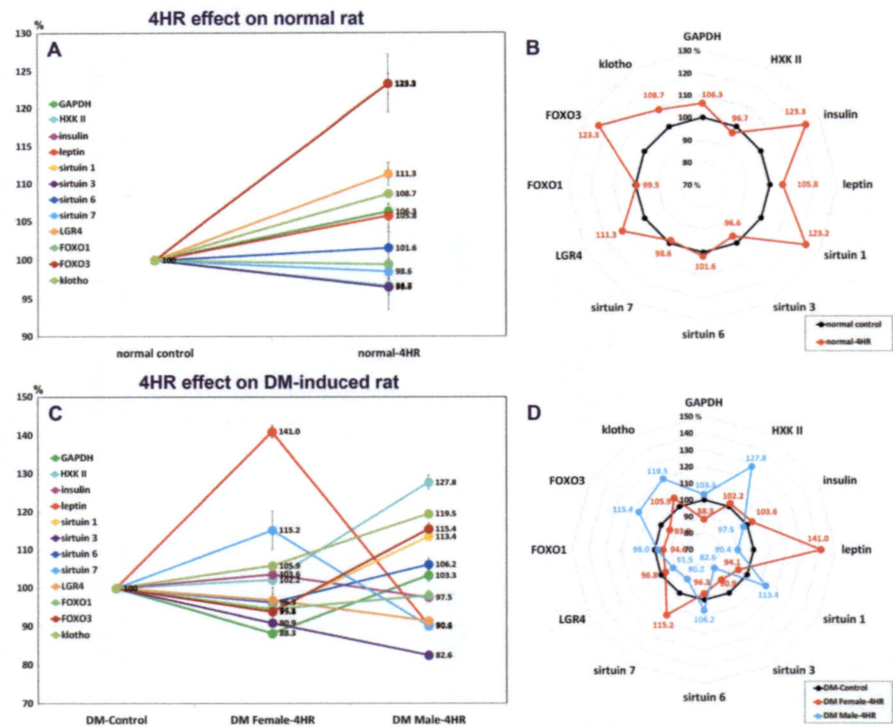

Fig. 8.6 Analysis of DM-related protein expression using IP-HPLC. (**a**) Line graph depicting the effects of 4HR on normal rats. (**b**) Star graph representation of the data in panel A. (**c**) Line graph illustrating the effects of 4HR on DM-induced female and male rats. (**d**) Star graph representation of the data in panel C

8.3 The Complication in Male Reproductive System

Diabetes can have a negative impact on the male reproductive system. Poorly controlled diabetes can cause various issues related to sexual and reproductive health in men [50]. Diabetes is one of the leading causes of erectile dysfunction [51]. High blood sugar levels can damage blood vessels and nerves, including those responsible for erections. This damage can reduce blood flow to the penis and impair nerve function, making it difficult to achieve or maintain an erection. Diabetes can also cause nerve damage that affects the muscles controlling the bladder and the release of semen during ejaculation [52]. This can lead to retrograde ejaculation, a condition in which semen enters the bladder instead of being expelled through the penis during ejaculation.

Men with diabetes may experience a decrease in sex drive due to hormonal imbalances, psychological factors such as anxiety or depression, or side effects from medications used to manage diabetes or its complications [53]. Diabetes, particularly type 2, has been associated with lower testosterone levels in men [54]. Low testosterone can contribute to erectile dysfunction, reduced libido, fatigue, and mood changes [55]. Diabetes can impact semen quality, including sperm count, motility, and morphology [56]. High blood sugar levels and oxidative stress can damage sperm DNA, potentially affecting fertility [56].

In this study, we prepared one testis from each animal and measured its weight. The average weight of the untreated control group was 1.15 ± 0.51 g, while the 4HR group had an average weight of 1.86 ± 0.26 g (Fig. 8.7a). The difference between the groups was statistically significant ($P = 0.002$). LGR4 is expressed in Sertoli cells, the supporting cells within the seminiferous tubules of the testes, which play a crucial role in spermatogenesis [57]. Studies have shown that loss of LGR4 function in mice leads to spermatogenesis defects, including disrupted Sertoli cell function, abnormal sperm morphology, and reduced sperm count [58]. The relative expression level of LGR4 in the untreated control group was 0.47 ± 0.11, while it was 0.89 ± 0.26 in the 4HR group (Fig. 8.7b). The difference between the groups was statistically significant ($P = 0.021$).

Upon histological examination, the untreated control group exhibited degeneration of Sertoli cells and Leydig cells (Fig. 8.7c). Additionally, abnormalities were observed in the tail portion of spermatocytes (Fig. 8.7c). These abnormalities could be attributed to impaired spermatogenesis due to the impact of diabetes on testicular structure and function [59]. Tail abnormalities can affect sperm motility, which is vital for sperm to swim and fertilize an egg, leading to reduced fertility in diabetic animals [59]. It is important to note that the severity and type of abnormalities may vary based on the specific animal model, diabetes duration, and severity. In contrast, the testes of the 4HR group displayed fewer abnormalities compared to the untreated control group (Fig. 8.7c), with no morphological abnormalities observed in spermatocytes. Due to the suppression of LGR4 expression in DM animals [58], the untreated control group exhibited a lower level of LGR4 expression in comparison to the 4HR group (Fig. 8.7c). This finding was consistent with the results of the Western blot analysis (Fig. 8.7b).

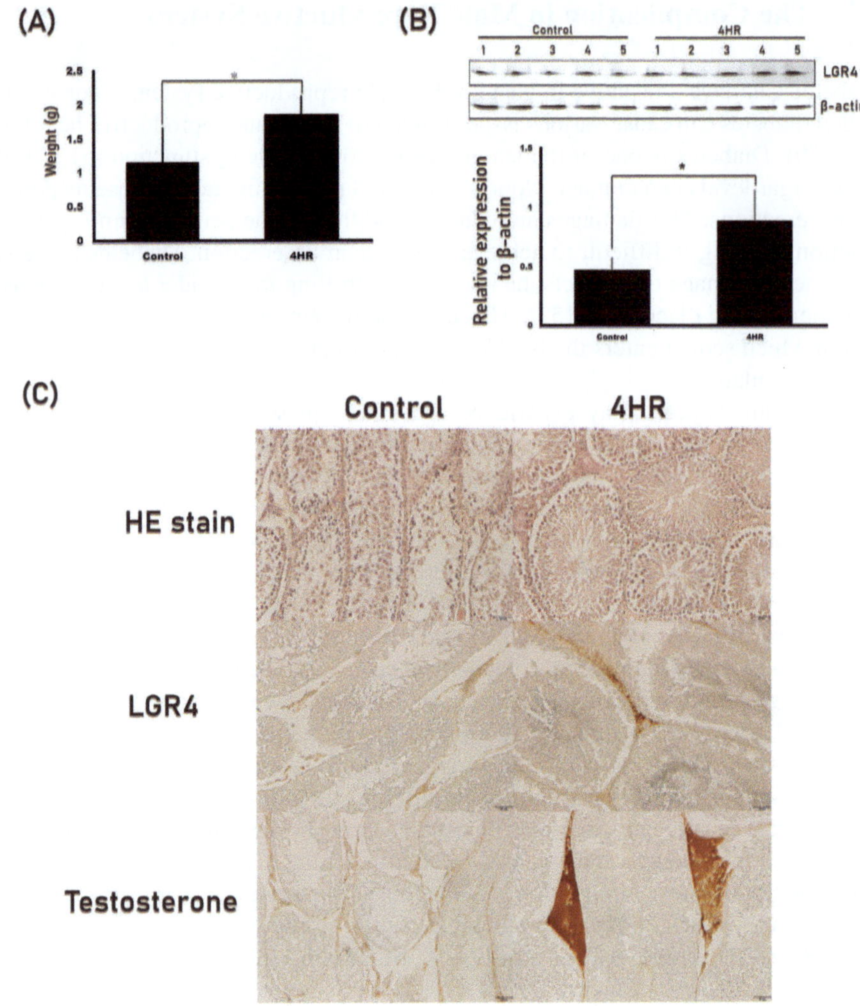

Fig. 8.7 Analysis of testes in the DM animal model. (**a**) Comparison of testes weight between groups. The weight of the 4HR group was significantly higher than that of the untreated control (*$P < 0.05$). (**b**) Western blot of LGR4 from tissue samples. The expression level of LGR4 was significantly higher in the 4HR group compared to the untreated control group (*$P < 0.05$). (**c**) Histological analysis. In the H&E stain, the spermatocytes of the untreated control group displayed poorly developed tail portions. However, spermatocytes in the 4HR group exhibited well-developed tail portions. Additionally, the expression levels of LGR4 and testosterone were higher in the 4HR group compared to the untreated control group

STZ-induced diabetes can negatively impact Leydig cell function, leading to a decrease in testosterone production [59]. As a result, the expression level of testosterone was lower in the untreated control group compared to the 4HR group (Fig. 8.7c). This finding contrasts with a previous publication [41]. The initial step of steroidogenesis, the conversion of cholesterol to pregnenolone, takes place in the mitochondria and is catalyzed by the enzyme cytochrome P450scc (cholesterol side-chain cleavage enzyme) [60]. Since 4HR is known to reduce mitochondrial function [4], its administration in healthy growing rats has been shown to decrease serum testosterone levels [41]. In previous experiments with growing healthy animals [41], the serum testosterone level of the untreated control was 10.19 ± 3.45 ng/mL, while it was 3.52 ± 1.05 ng/mL in the 4HR group. In this study, the serum testosterone level of the untreated control was 2.92 ± 0.08 ng/mL, and 3.23 ± 0.19 ng/mL in the 4HR group. Although the serum testosterone level of the DM-4HR group was higher than that of the DM-untreated control group, it remained lower than that of the healthy-4HR group. The serum testosterone level in rats can exhibit high variations depending on the time of collection, even within the same animal [61]. Therefore, the serum testosterone level should be considered as a reference.

Interestingly, the administration of 4HR significantly decreased the count of apoptotic cells within the testis (Fig. 8.8), typically heightened in diabetic conditions [62, 63]. This aligns with other research where the administration of insulin in type 1 DM decreased the count of p53-positive cells within the testis [63]. This study suggests that 4HR may alleviate the increase in apoptotic cells within the testis induced by diabetes, further protecting testicular function.

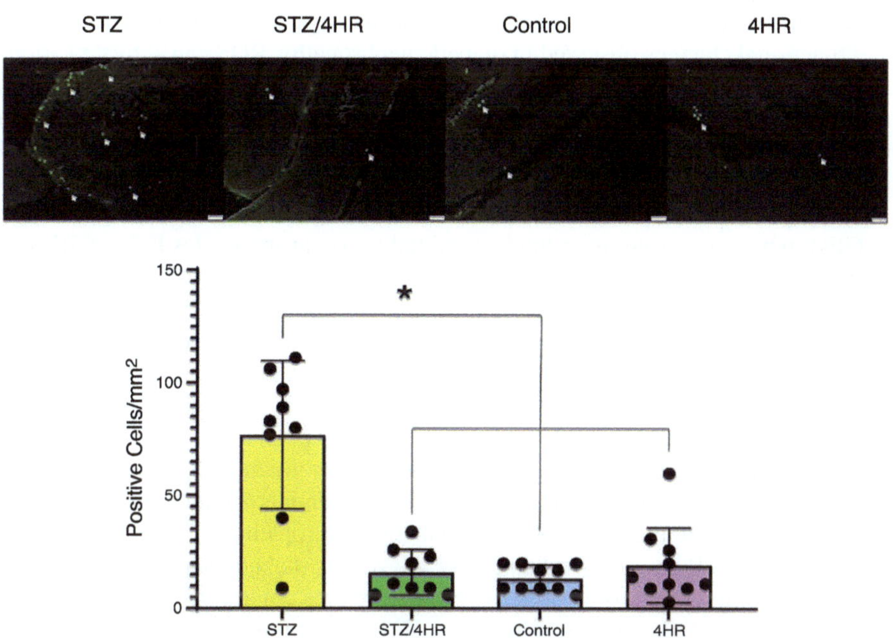

Fig. 8.8 The quantification of TUNEL-positive cells per square millimeter. The STZ group exhibited a considerably higher count of TUNEL-positive cells in comparison to the other groups (*$p < 0.001$)

8.4 The Complication in the Kidney

Diabetic nephropathy, a kidney-related complication of diabetes, arises from the damaging effects of high blood sugar levels on the kidneys' delicate blood vessels [64]. Persistent high blood sugar levels can damage the small blood vessels in the kidneys, impairing their ability to filter waste products and ultimately leading to kidney failure in severe cases [65]. Both type 1 and type 2 diabetes patients with suboptimal blood sugar control and elevated blood pressure are more susceptible to diabetic nephropathy.

Diabetic nephropathy has been linked to ROS [66]. ROS are chemically reactive molecules containing oxygen, which are generated as a natural by-product of cellular metabolism [67]. Under normal conditions, ROS play a role in cellular signaling and the immune response [68]. However, when ROS production exceeds the body's antioxidant defense mechanisms, oxidative stress occurs [68]. Oxidative stress can damage cellular components, including proteins, lipids, and DNA, leading to cellular dysfunction and tissue injury [69]. In the context of diabetes, chronically elevated blood sugar levels contribute to the increased production of ROS and oxidative stress [66].

Excessive ROS can cause direct injury to the kidney cells, including podocytes, mesangial cells, and endothelial cells [70]. This damage contributes to the structural and functional changes observed in diabetic nephropathy. ROS can activate various signaling pathways, such as the mitogen-activated protein kinase (MAPK) pathway, nuclear factor-kappa B (NF-κB) pathway, and transforming growth factor-beta (TGF-β) pathway [71]. These pathways are involved in inflammation, fibrosis, and cell death, which contribute to kidney damage in diabetic nephropathy. Elevated blood sugar levels promote the formation of advanced glycation end products (AGEs), which are proteins or lipids modified by sugar molecules [72]. AGEs can bind to their receptor (RAGE) and stimulate the production of ROS, further exacerbating oxidative stress and promoting inflammation and fibrosis in the kidneys [73]. Diabetes can also impair the body's natural antioxidant defense mechanisms, reducing its ability to neutralize ROS and making the kidneys more susceptible to oxidative damage [74].

Targeting oxidative stress has been proposed as a potential therapeutic strategy for diabetic nephropathy. Antioxidant agents, such as vitamin E, alpha-lipoic acid, and N-acetylcysteine, have been studied for their potential to reduce oxidative stress and prevent or slow the progression of diabetic nephropathy [75]. 4HR is antioxidant agent [76, 77] and may be helpful for alleviating diabetic nephropathy.

PAS staining is commonly used to detect structures containing polysaccharides, glycoproteins, and glycolipids in histological tissue samples [78]. In the context of diabetic nephropathy, PAS staining can highlight certain pathological changes in the kidney, such as the thickening of the glomerular basement membrane and the accumulation of extracellular matrix material in the mesangial area [79]. These changes are typically associated with the progression of diabetic nephropathy. Therefore, it is common to observe PAS-positive staining in kidney tissue samples from diabetic individuals or animals with diabetic nephropathy [79].

In our study, kidney tissue samples from the untreated control group demonstrated strong PAS-positive staining (Fig. 8.9). However, kidney tissue samples from the 4HR group displayed weaker PAS staining compared to the untreated control group (Fig. 8.9). Consequently, the histological sections predominantly exhibited counterstaining, such as hematoxylin and light green (Fig. 8.9). Tumor necrosis factor-α (TNF-α) serves as an inflammation marker, and the glomeruli of diabetic kidneys present high TNF-α expression levels [80]. In this study, the glomeruli of the untreated control group revealed high TNF-α expression levels (Fig. 8.10). In contrast, the 4HR group's TNF-α expression levels were lower than those of the untreated control group (Fig. 8.9). 4HR has been shown to inhibit TNF-α expression in burn wounds [81] and suppress the NF-κB pathway [82, 83]. Therefore, 4HR might inhibit TNF-α expression by inhibiting the NF-κB pathway. Interestingly, we observed a similar pattern of findings in the liver samples (Fig. 8.10).

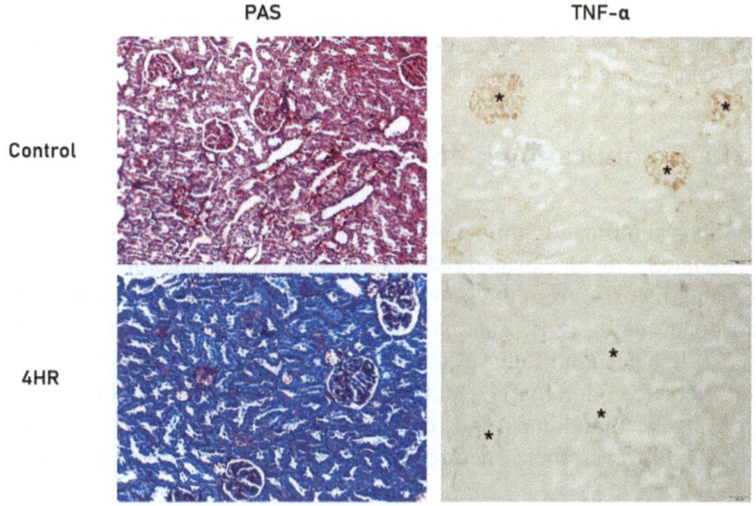

Fig. 8.9 Evaluation of kidney tissue in the DM animal model. The untreated control group displayed a strong positive reaction to PAS staining, as indicated by the intense deep pink color. In contrast, the 4HR group exhibited a weaker positive reaction to PAS staining, as evidenced by the background staining. Notably, the glomeruli (asterisks) in the untreated control group showed a strong positive reaction to tumor necrosis factor-α (TNF-α) immunostaining. However, the glomeruli (asterisks) in the 4HR group were negative for TNF-α immunostaining (original magnification ×200)

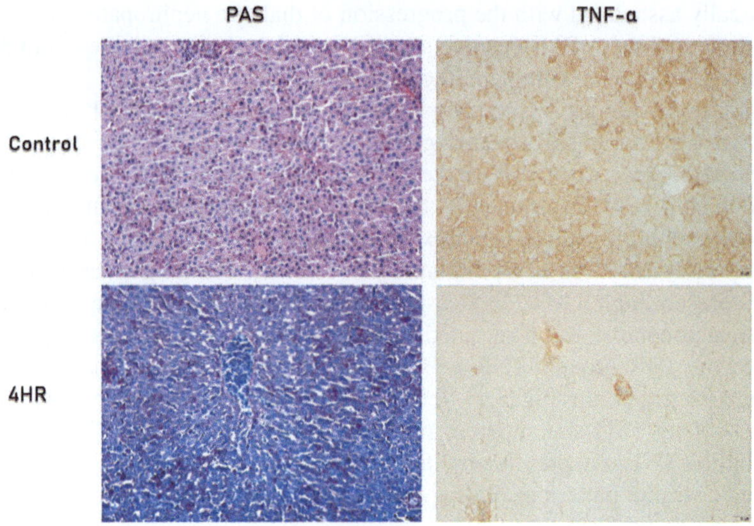

Fig. 8.10 Evaluation of liver tissue in the DM animal model: The untreated control group exhibited a strong positive reaction to PAS staining in comparison to the 4HR group. Additionally, the untreated control group demonstrated a strong positive reaction to tumor necrosis factor-α (TNF-α) immunostaining (original magnification ×200)

8.5 The Complication in the Bone

Bone health is significantly influenced by DM, with both type 1 and type 2 diabetes being associated with an elevated risk of bone-related complications. These complications primarily arise from the impact of diabetes on bone metabolism, bone density, and bone quality [84]. Extensive research has demonstrated that individuals with type 1 diabetes tend to have lower bone mineral density (BMD) compared to their non-diabetic counterparts, resulting in an increased susceptibility to fractures [85]. Conversely, individuals with type 2 diabetes might exhibit normal or even higher BMD; however, their fracture risk remains elevated due to diminished bone quality [86].

The alteration of bone metabolism in individuals with diabetes is likely attributed to a variety of factors. Chronic hyperglycemia, a hallmark of diabetes, impairs osteoblast (bone-forming cells) function and promotes osteoclast (bone-resorbing cells) activity, leading to a decrease in bone formation and an increase in bone resorption. Additionally, diabetic individuals may experience hormonal imbalances, such as deficiencies in insulin and growth hormone, which further contribute to disturbed bone metabolism. These disturbances ultimately result in an imbalance between bone formation and resorption, leading to compromised bone health.

The implications of impaired bone health in individuals with diabetes are clinically significant. The increased risk of fractures observed in type 1 diabetes highlights the importance of early identification and intervention to prevent skeletal complications. In type 2 diabetes, where BMD may be preserved or slightly elevated, attention should be directed toward assessing bone quality through techniques such as bone microarchitecture analysis and assessing fracture risk based on factors beyond BMD. Strategies to improve bone health in individuals with diabetes may include optimizing glycemic control, ensuring adequate intake of bone-supportive nutrients such as calcium and vitamin D, and promoting weight-bearing exercises to enhance bone strength. Moreover, close collaboration between endocrinologists and orthopedic specialists is vital to provide comprehensive care and reduce the burden of bone-related complications in individuals with diabetes.

Diabetes can negatively affect bone quality through various mechanisms, such as increased inflammation, oxidative stress, accumulation of AGEs, and impaired collagen synthesis [87]. These factors can lead to weakened bone structure and increased fracture risk. Diabetes can disrupt bone metabolism, affecting the balance between bone formation and resorption. In type 1 diabetes, there is usually a reduction in bone formation due to the lack of insulin's anabolic effects on bone [84]. In type 2 diabetes, the situation is more complex, with both bone formation and resorption potentially affected, leading to impaired bone remodeling [84]. Some diabetes-related complications, such as neuropathy, can increase the risk of falls and fractures, while poor blood circulation can impair the bone healing process [88].

The impact of 4HR administration on bone was assessed using μCT analysis of femur samples. The average cortical bone thickness was 0.58 ± 0.03 mm in the healthy group and 0.36 ± 0.05 mm in the DM group. This difference between the groups was statistically significant ($P < 0.001$). No significant difference was observed between the untreated control group and the 4HR group in healthy animals ($P > 0.05$). However, a significant difference was found between the untreated control group and the 4HR group in DM animals ($P = 0.001$). The average cortical bone thickness measured 0.33 ± 0.04 mm in the untreated group and 0.39 ± 0.04 mm in the 4HR group (Fig. 8.11).

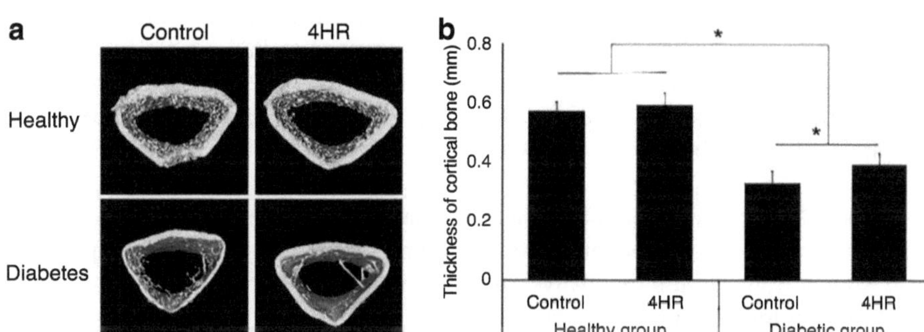

Fig. 8.11 Assessment of femur in the DM animal model. (**a**) Micro-computerized tomography (μCT) analysis reveals the cross-sectional image of the femur. The cross-sectional area is generally smaller in the DM group compared to the healthy group. Notably, the cortical bone thickness in the untreated control of the DM group is the thinnest among all groups. (**b**) Cortical bone thickness comparisons among the groups show that the DM group has significantly lower thickness compared to the healthy group (*$P < 0.05$). Within the DM group, the 4HR group exhibits significantly greater thickness compared to the untreated control group (*$P < 0.05$)

The exact mechanism of 4HR on the bone of diabetic animal has not been clarified. Potential mechanism can be suggested as follows. 4HR may help reduce inflammation in diabetic animals, which could promote a healthier bone microenvironment. By suppressing pro-inflammatory cytokines, such as TNF-α [81], 4HR may positively influence bone remodeling processes and improve bone formation. 4HR may have antioxidant effects that help neutralize ROS and combat oxidative stress [76, 77]. Oxidative stress is known to impair bone health in diabetes [89]. By reducing oxidative stress, 4HR may help preserve bone integrity and promote bone formation. 4HR may directly or indirectly influence the balance between bone formation and bone resorption, either by promoting osteoblast activity (bone-building cells) [41] or inhibiting osteoclast activity (bone-resorbing cells) [82], leading to increased cortical bone thickness in diabetic animals. Further research would be needed to confirm the exact mechanism through which 4HR administration increases cortical bone thickness in a DM animal model.

8.6 The Complication in the Tasting

Numerous studies have found that people with DM have altered taste thresholds. These individuals often exhibit changes in their ability to perceive tastes, such as hydrochloric acid, sucrose, sodium chloride, and urea [32, 33]. Electrogustometric measurements have shown that the taste threshold for electrical stimulation can vary widely in people with diabetes compared to healthy individuals [90, 91]. This indicates a potential disruption in the normal functioning of taste receptors and transduction pathways. DM often causes sensory deficits that manifest in various ways, including taste disorders. These taste alterations can occur early in the disease course and may be generalized across different taste modalities.

Although not explicitly linked to apoptosis in the available literature, diabetes has been associated with morphological changes in taste buds in animal studies, such as those using streptozotocin-induced diabetic rats [92]. Taste disorders can have a profound impact on quality of life, affecting dietary choices, nutritional status, and even metabolic control, which is particularly relevant for individuals with DM.

While the exact molecular mechanisms remain underexplored, some studies suggest that changes in taste receptor expression and function, as well as disruptions in taste signal transduction pathways, may be involved. For example, G-protein-coupled receptors like gustducin could be affected in the context of DM [93].

In the taste bud analysis, the TUNEL assay revealed significant differences among the groups being investigated [94]. Within the DM group, there was a substantial decline in TUNEL-positive cells following 4HR treatment compared to the untreated control group ($*P < 0.05$; Fig. 8.12). Upon examining selected microscopic images, it became evident that the control group had a greater number of cells undergoing apoptosis than the 4HR group (Fig. 8.12). This suggests that 4HR

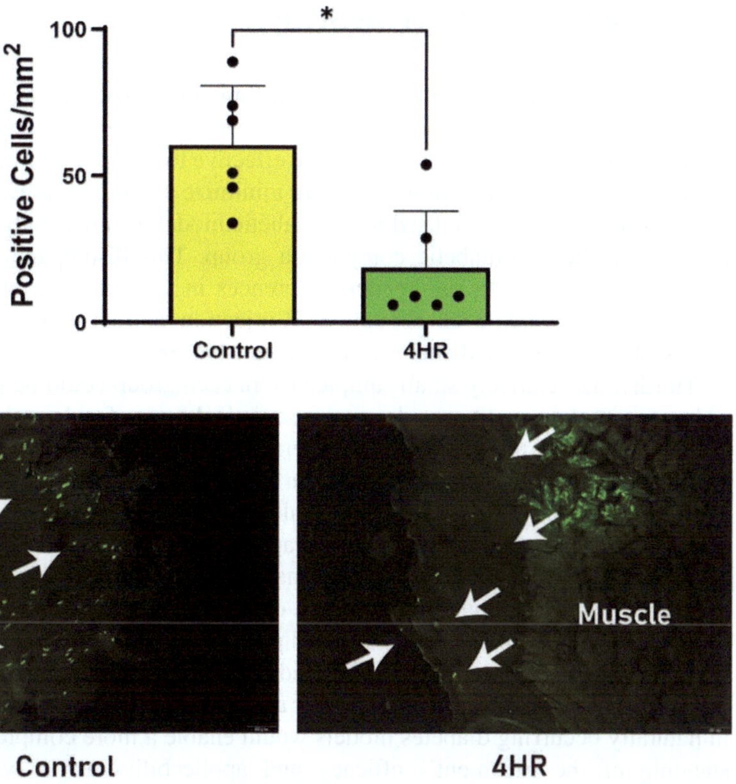

Fig. 8.12 The results from the terminal deoxynucleotidyl transferase dUTP nick end labeling (TUNEL) assay revealed significant differences between the studied groups. Within the context of the DM group, the 4HR group exhibited a significantly lower number of TUNEL positive cells compared to the untreated control group (*$P < 0.05$). Upon visual examination of selected images, it was evident that TUNEL positive nuclei, as indicated by the presence of labeling, were more prominently observed in the control group compared to the 4HR group

treatment could be effective in diminishing apoptosis. The data strongly associate 4HR treatment with reduced apoptosis in the diabetic tongue, notably in the epithelial layer. The pronounced disparity between the control and 4HR groups underscores the potential effectiveness of this treatment in mitigating epithelial cell death. It should be noted, however, that due to the limitations of the animal study, the difference in taste perception was not assessed.

Grasping the influence of DM on taste sensitivity is essential for better managing and treating this medical condition, especially considering the importance of dietary control in diabetes management. Upcoming studies that focus on specialized interventions—such as the employment of chemical chaperones to avert apoptosis in taste buds—could offer valuable insights into alleviating the taste-related complications commonly associated with DM.

8.7 Limitation of Current Study

Our current animal study presents several limitations that should be addressed in future research. Firstly, although blinding techniques were employed during data collection and analysis, it would be more effective to ensure blinding during animal grouping and treatment administration to minimize potential biases. Secondly, both male and female rats were used in the diabetic model, whereas only male rats were included in the non-diabetic comparison group. This discrepancy may limit the interpretation of results, as gender differences in treatment responses cannot be adequately assessed, even though STZ-injection animal models are generally unsuitable for inducing diabetes in female rats [95, 96].

Thirdly, the relatively small sample size in each group could be improved upon, as larger samples would provide greater statistical power for detecting group differences and reduce the risk of Type II errors (failing to detect a genuine effect). Fourthly, using only one 4HR dosage in the experimental group limits the study, incorporating multiple dosage levels would better assess the dose-response relationship and help determine the optimal therapeutic dose.

Fifthly, the 12-week study duration may be insufficient for evaluating the long-term effects and potential complications of the treatments. A more extended study duration or follow-up assessments could provide deeper insights into the interventions' long-term impacts. Lastly, the study relies on a single animal model (STZ-induced diabetes in rats). Including other animal models or examining the treatment in naturally occurring diabetes models would enable a more comprehensive understanding of the treatment's efficacy and applicability across various diabetic conditions.

8.8 Closing Remark

The effects of administering 4HR were examined in both healthy animal models and STZ-induced DM animal models in this chapter. The benefits of 4HR administration in terms of bone biology in healthy animals were not clear. However, definite benefits were observed in the STZ-induced DM animal model, including a decrease in blood sugar levels through potential increases in GLUT expression in the liver, alleviation of DM-induced weight loss, prevention of DM-induced abnormality in the testes, and alleviation of diabetic nephropathy and cortical bone loss. Nonetheless, the current study had several limitations, as mentioned in the preceding section. Given the significant interest in DM, further research is necessary.

Acknowledgments The IP-HPLC experiment was conducted, and its results were interpreted by Professor Suk Keun Lee, who belongs to the Institution of Hydrogen Magnetic Reaction Gene Regulation in Korea. Additionally, Professor Lee kindly reviewed this chapter. On the other hand, Professor Dae-Won Kim from Gangneung-Wonju National University in Korea carried out the Western blot in the tissue sample and performed the assay using serum.

References

1. Allen JF (2015) Why chloroplasts and mitochondria retain their own genomes and genetic systems: colocation for redox regulation of gene expression. Proc Natl Acad Sci USA 112:10231–10238
2. Gray MW, Burger G, Lang BF (1999) Mitochondrial evolution. Science 283:1476–1481
3. Nikolaev YA, Tutel'yan AV, Loiko NG et al (2020) The use of 4-hexylresorcinol as antibiotic adjuvant. PLoS One 15:e0239147
4. Hernansanz-Agustín P, Enríquez JA (2021) Generation of reactive oxygen species by mitochondria. Antioxidants (Basel) 10:415
5. Rueda EM, Johnson JE Jr, Giddabasappa A et al (2016) The cellular and compartmental profile of mouse retinal glycolysis, tricarboxylic acid cycle, oxidative phosphorylation, and ~P transferring kinases. Mol Vis 22:847–885
6. Kwak SH, Park KS, Lee KU, Lee HK (2010) Mitochondrial metabolism and diabetes. J Diabetes Investig 1:161–169
7. Yang L, Mih N, Anand A et al (2019) Cellular responses to reactive oxygen species are predicted from molecular mechanisms. Proc Natl Acad Sci USA 116:14368–14373
8. Newsholme P, Cruzat VF, Keane KN, Carlessi R, de Bittencourt PI Jr (2016) Molecular mechanisms of ROS production and oxidative stress in diabetes. Biochem J 473:4527–4550
9. Andreadi A, Bellia A, Di Daniele N et al (2022) The molecular link between oxidative stress, insulin resistance, and type 2 diabetes: a target for new therapies against cardiovascular diseases. Curr Opin Pharmacol 62:85–96
10. Eguchi N, Vaziri ND, Dafoe DC, Ichii H (2021) The role of oxidative stress in pancreatic β cell dysfunction in diabetes. Int J Mol Sci 22:1509
11. Rovira-Llopis S, Bañuls C, Diaz-Morales N et al (2017) Mitochondrial dynamics in type 2 diabetes: pathophysiological implications. Redox Biol 11:637–645
12. Fealy CE, Mulya A, Axelrod CL, Kirwan JP (2018) Mitochondrial dynamics in skeletal muscle insulin resistance and type 2 diabetes. Transl Res 202:69–82
13. Santos JM, Tewari S, Goldberg AF, Kowluru RA (2011) Mitochondrial biogenesis and the development of diabetic retinopathy. Free Radic Biol Med 51(10):1849–1860
14. Singh R, Mohapatra L, Tripathi AS (2021) Targeting mitochondrial biogenesis: a potential approach for preventing and controlling diabetes. Futur J Pharm Sci 7:212
15. Ramakrishna MP, Pavithran PV, Bhavani N et al (2019) Mitochondrial diabetes: more than just hyperglycemia. Clin Diabetes 37(3):298–301
16. He Q, Ma P, Torshizi R (2022) The impact of some natural phenolic compounds on α-glucosidase and sorbitol dehydrogenase enzymes, and anti-leukemia cancer potential, spin density distributions, and in silico studies. J Oleo Sci 71(6):863–873
17. Kim SG (2020) Use of 4-hexylresorcinol for treating metabolic diseases and liver diseases. KR Patent 1020200133331
18. Zhu X, Jin C, Pan Q, Hu X (2021) Determining the quantitative relationship between glycolysis and GAPDH in cancer cells exhibiting the Warburg effect. J Biol Chem 296:100369
19. Zhao B, Qiang L, Joseph J, Kalyanaraman B, Viollet B, He YY (2016) Mitochondrial dysfunction activates the AMPK signaling and autophagy to promote cell survival. Genes Dis 3(1):82–87
20. Habegger KM, Hoffman NJ, Ridenour CM, Brozinick JT, Elmendorf JS (2012) AMPK enhances insulin-stimulated GLUT4 regulation via lowering membrane cholesterol. Endocrinology 153(5):2130–2141
21. Soyoye DO, Abiodun OO, Ikem RT, Kolawole BA, Akintomide AO (2021) Diabetes and peripheral artery disease: a review. World J Diabetes 12(6):827–838
22. Kumsa HT, Abdisa LG, Tolessa LT et al (2023) Early detection and treatment device for diabetic foot neuropathy. Ir J Med Sci 192(1):143–148

23. Orlando G, Balducci S, Boulton AJM, Degens H, Reeves ND (2022) Neuromuscular dysfunction and exercise training in people with diabetic peripheral neuropathy: a narrative review. Diabetes Res Clin Pract 183:109183
24. Sagoo MK, Gnudi L (2020) Diabetic nephropathy: an overview. Methods Mol Biol 2067:3–7
25. Mohite AA, Perais JA, McCullough P, Lois N (2023) Retinal ischaemia in diabetic retinopathy: understanding and overcoming a therapeutic challenge. J Clin Med 12(6):2406
26. Brekelmans W, van Laar W, Tolen NJ, Hoencamp R, Borger van der Burg BLS (2023) Recurrent diabetic foot ulcers: results of a maximal multidisciplinary approach including reconstructive foot/ankle surgery. Int Wound J 20:1866. https://doi.org/10.1111/iwj.14045
27. de Macedo GM, Nunes S, Barreto T (2016) Skin disorders in diabetes mellitus: an epidemiology and physiopathology review. Diabetol Metab Syndr 8(1):63
28. Gioacchini FM, Pisani D, Viola P et al (2023) Diabetes mellitus and hearing loss: a complex relationship. Medicina (Kaunas) 59(2):269
29. Tanriover C, Ucku D, Akyol M et al (2023) Potential use of SGLT-2 inhibitors in obstructive sleep apnea: a new treatment on the horizon. Sleep Breath 27(1):77–89
30. Arsh A, Afaq S, Carswell C, Bhatti MM, Ullah I, Siddiqi N (2023) Effectiveness of physical activity in managing co-morbid depression in adults with type 2 diabetes mellitus: a systematic review and meta-analysis. J Affect Disord 329:448–459
31. Soliman H, Gourcerol G (2023) Targeting the pylorus in gastroparesis: from physiology to endoscopic pyloromyotomy. Neurogastroenterol Motil 35(2):e14529
32. Pugnaloni S, Alia S, Mancini M et al (2020) A study on the relationship between type 2 diabetes and taste function in patients with good glycemic control. Nutrients 12(4):1112
33. Reiter ER, DiNardo LJ, Costanzo RM (2006) Toxic effects on gustatory function. Adv Otorhinolaryngol 63:265–277
34. Perona JS (2017) Membrane lipid alterations in the metabolic syndrome and the role of dietary oils. Biochim Biophys Acta Biomembr 1859(9 Pt B):1690-1703:1690
35. Yu J, Sharma P, Girgis CM, Gunton JE (2022) Vitamin D and beta cells in type 1 diabetes: a systematic review. Int J Mol Sci 23(22):14434
36. Petroni ML, Brodosi L, Marchignoli F et al (2021) Nutrition in patients with type 2 diabetes: present knowledge and remaining challenges. Nutrients 13(8):2748
37. Pereira RO, Wende AR, Olsen C et al (2013) Inducible overexpression of GLUT1 prevents mitochondrial dysfunction and attenuates structural remodeling in pressure overload but does not prevent left ventricular dysfunction. J Am Heart Assoc 2(5):e000301
38. Kahn BB (1998) Type 2 diabetes: when insulin secretion fails to compensate for insulin resistance. Cell 92(5):593–596
39. American Diabetes Association (2019) Classification and diagnosis of diabetes: standards of medical care in diabetes-2019. Diabetes Care 42(Suppl 1):S13–S28
40. Vallon V, Thomson SC (2020) The tubular hypothesis of nephron filtration and diabetic kidney disease. Nat Rev Nephrol 16(6):317–336
41. Lee IS, Kim DW, Oh JH et al (2021) Effects of 4-hexylresorcinol on craniofacial growth in rats. Int J Mol Sci 22(16):8935
42. Mueckler M, Thorens B (2013) The SLC2 (GLUT) family of membrane transporters. Mol Asp Med 34(2–3):121–138
43. Simpson IA, Dwyer D, Malide D, Moley KH, Travis A, Vannucci SJ (2008) The facilitative glucose transporter GLUT3: 20 years of distinction. Am J Physiol Endocrinol Metab 295(2):E242–E253
44. Thorens B, Mueckler M (2010) Glucose transporters in the 21st century. Am J Physiol Endocrinol Metab 298(2):E141–E145
45. Klip A, McGraw TE, James DE (2019) Thirty sweet years of GLUT4. J Biol Chem 294(30):11369–11381
46. Petersen MC, Shulman GI (2018) Mechanisms of insulin action and insulin resistance. Physiol Rev 98(4):2133–2223
47. Thorens B (2015) GLUT2, glucose sensing and glucose homeostasis. Diabetologia 58(2):221–232

48. Yki-Järvinen H (2004) Thiazolidinediones. N Engl J Med 351(11):1106–1118
49. Lehmann JM, Moore LB, Smith-Oliver TA, Wilkison WO, Willson TM, Kliewer SA (1995) An antidiabetic thiazolidinedione is a high affinity ligand for peroxisome proliferator-activated receptor gamma (PPAR gamma). J Biol Chem 270(22):12953–12956
50. Maiorino MI, Bellastella G, Esposito K (2014) Diabetes and sexual dysfunction: current perspectives. Diabetes Metab Syndr Obes 7:95–105
51. Hackett G (2009) Diabetic impotence. In: Mulhall JP, Hedges JC (eds) Textbook of erectile dysfunction. Informa Healthcare, London, pp 183–194
52. Yafi FA, Jenkins L, Albersen M et al (2016) Erectile dysfunction. Nat Rev Dis Primers 2:16003
53. Malavige LS, Levy JC (2009) Erectile dysfunction in diabetes mellitus. J Sex Med 6(5):1232–1247
54. Dhindsa S, Prabhakar S, Sethi M, Bandyopadhyay A, Chaudhuri A, Dandona P (2004) Frequent occurrence of hypogonadotropic hypogonadism in type 2 diabetes. J Clin Endocrinol Metab 89(11):5462–5468
55. Traish AM, Miner MM, Morgentaler A, Zitzmann M (2011) Testosterone deficiency. Am J Med 124(7):578–587
56. La Vignera S, Condorelli RA, Di Mauro M et al (2015) Reproductive function in male patients with type 1 diabetes mellitus. Andrology 3(6):1082–1087
57. Song H, Luo J, Luo W et al (2008) Inactivation of G-protein-coupled receptor 48 (Gpr48/Lgr4) impairs definitive erythropoiesis at midgestation through down-regulation of the ATF4 signaling pathway. J Biol Chem 283(52):36687–36697
58. Mendive F, Laurent P, Van Schoore G, Skarnes W, Pochet R, Vassart G (2006) Defective postnatal development of the male reproductive tract in LGR4 knockout mice. Dev Biol 290(2):421–434
59. Navarro-Casado L, Juncos-Tobarra MA, Cháfer-Rudilla M, de Onzoño LÍ, Blázquez-Cabrera JA, Miralles-García JM (2010) Effect of experimental diabetes and STZ on male fertility capacity. Study in rats. J Androl 31(6):584–592
60. Miller WL, Auchus RJ (2011) The molecular biology, biochemistry, and physiology of human steroidogenesis and its disorders. Endocr Rev 32:81–151
61. Gao W, Stalder T, Foley P, Rauh M, Deng H, Kirschbaum C (2013) Quantitative analysis of steroid hormones in human hair using a column-switching LC-APCI-MS/MS assay. J Chromatogr B Analyt Technol Biomed Life Sci 928:1–8
62. Nna VU, Abu Bakar AB, Ahmad A, Eleazu CO, Mohamed M (2019) Oxidative stress, NF-κB-mediated inflammation and apoptosis in the testes of streptozotocin-induced diabetic rats: combined protective effects of Malaysian propolis and metformin. Antioxidants 8(10):465
63. Minas A, Talebi H, Taravat Ray M, Yari Eisalou M, Alves MG, Razi M (2021) Insulin treatment to type 1 male diabetic rats protects fertility by avoiding testicular apoptosis and cell cycle arrest. Gene 799:145847
64. Alicic RZ, Rooney MT, Tuttle KR (2017) Diabetic kidney disease: challenges, progress, and possibilities. Clin J Am Soc Nephrol 12:2032–2045
65. Tonneijck L, Muskiet MH, Smits MM et al (2017) Glomerular hyperfiltration in diabetes: mechanisms, clinical significance, and treatment. J Am Soc Nephrol 28:1023–1039
66. Forbes JM, Cooper ME (2013) Mechanisms of diabetic complications. Physiol Rev 93:137–188
67. Lambeth JD (2004) NOX enzymes and the biology of reactive oxygen. Nat Rev Immunol 4:181–189
68. Sies H (2015) Oxidative stress: a concept in redox biology and medicine. Redox Biol 4:180–183
69. Poljsak B, Milisav I (2012) The neglected significance of "antioxidative stress". Oxidative Med Cell Longev 2012:480895
70. Jha JC, Banal C, Chow BS, Cooper ME, Jandeleit-Dahm K (2016) Diabetes and kidney disease: role of oxidative stress. Antioxid Redox Signal 25:657–684
71. Finkel T, Holbrook NJ (2000) Oxidants, oxidative stress and the biology of ageing. Nature 408:239–247
72. Singh R, Barden A, Mori T, Beilin L (2001) Advanced glycation end-products: a review. Diabetologia 44:129–146

73. Yamagishi S, Imaizumi T (2005) Diabetic vascular complications: pathophysiology, biochemical basis and potential therapeutic strategy. Curr Pharm Des 11:2279–2299
74. Brownlee M (2005) The pathobiology of diabetic complications: a unifying mechanism. Diabetes 54:1615–1625
75. Papadimitriou A, Peixoto EB, Silva KC, Lopes de Faria JM, Lopes de Faria JB (2014) Increase in AMPK brought about by cocoa is renoprotective in experimental diabetes mellitus by reducing NOX4/TGFβ-1 signaling. J Nutr Biochem 25:773–784
76. Jo YY, Kim DW, Choi JY, Kim SG (2019) 4-hexylresorcinol and silk sericin increase the expression of vascular endothelial growth factor via different pathways. Sci Rep 9:3448
77. Yen GC, Duh PD, Lin CW (2003) Effects of resveratrol and 4-hexylresorcinol on hydrogen peroxide-induced oxidative DNA damage in human lymphocytes. Free Radic Res 37:509–514
78. McManus JF (1948) Histological and histochemical uses of periodic acid. Stain Technol 23:99–108
79. Susztak K, Raff AC, Schiffer M, Böttinger EP (2006) Glucose-induced reactive oxygen species cause apoptosis of podocytes and podocyte depletion at the onset of diabetic nephropathy. Diabetes 55:225–233
80. Chow F, Ozols E, Nikolic-Paterson DJ, Atkins RC, Tesch GH (2004) Macrophages in mouse type 2 diabetic nephropathy: correlation with diabetic state and progressive renal injury. Kidney Int 65:116–128
81. Ahn J, Kim SG, Kim MK et al (2016) Topical delivery of 4-hexylresorcinol promotes wound healing via tumor necrosis factor-α suppression. Burns 42:1534–1541
82. Song JY, Kim SG, Park NR, Choi JY (2018) Porcine bone incorporated with 4-hexylresorcinol increases new bone formation by suppression of the nuclear factor kappa B signaling pathway. J Craniofac Surg 29:1983–1990
83. Yi W, Liu T, Gao X, Xie Y, Liu M (2021) 4-hexylresorcinol inhibits osteoclastogenesis by suppressing the NF-κB signaling pathway and reverses bone loss in ovariectomized mice. Exp Ther Med 21:354
84. Napoli N, Chandran M, Pierroz DD et al (2017) Mechanisms of diabetes mellitus-induced bone fragility. Nat Rev Endocrinol 13:208–219
85. Shah VN, Shah CS, Snell-Bergeon JK (2015) Type 1 diabetes and risk of fracture: meta-analysis and review of the literature. Diabet Med 32:1134–1142
86. Vestergaard P (2007) Discrepancies in bone mineral density and fracture risk in patients with type 1 and type 2 diabetes—a meta-analysis. Osteoporos Int 18:427–444
87. Saito M, Marumo K (2010) Collagen cross-links as a determinant of bone quality: a possible explanation for bone fragility in aging, osteoporosis, and diabetes mellitus. Osteoporos Int 21:195–214
88. Schwartz AV, Sellmeyer DE (2007) Diabetes, fracture, and bone fragility. Curr Osteoporos Rep 5:105–111
89. Hamada Y, Fujii H, Fukagawa M (2009) Role of oxidative stress in diabetic bone disorder. Bone 45(Suppl 1):S35–S38
90. Le Floch JP, Le Lièvre G, Verroust J, Philippon C, Peynegre R, Perlemuter L (1990) Factors related to the electric taste threshold in type 1 diabetic patients. Diabet Med 7(6):526–531
91. Le Floch JP, Le Lièvre G, Labroue M, Paul M, Peynegre R, Perlemuter L (1993) Smell dysfunction and related factors in diabetic patients. Diabetes Care 16(6):934–937
92. Pai MH, Ko TL, Chou HC (2007) Effects of streptozotocin-induced diabetes on taste buds in rat vallate papillae. Acta Histochem 109(3):200–207
93. Zhou LH, Liu XM, Feng XH, Han LO, Liu GD (2009) Expression of alpha-gustducin in the circumvallate papillae of taste buds of diabetic rats. Acta Histochem 111(2):145–149
94. Gaida D, Park YW, Kim SG (2023) 4-hexylresorcinol and its effects on circumvallate papillae taste buds in diabetic and healthy rats: an initial investigation. Appl Sci 13(21):11617
95. Furman BL (2021) Streptozotocin-induced diabetic models in mice and rats. Curr Protoc 1:e78
96. Deeds MC, Anderson JM, Armstrong AS, Gastineau DA, Hiddinga HJ, Jahangir A, Eberhardt NL, Kudva YC (2011) Single dose streptozotocin-induced diabetes: considerations for study design in islet transplantation models. Lab Anim 45(3):131–140

Chapter 9
Limitations and Future Directions for 4-Hexylresorcinol Applications

Abstract This chapter explores the potential applications of 4-hexylresorcinol (4HR) in various medical fields, including neurologic disease, dental pulp regeneration, viral disease, and osteoporosis. 4HR is an organic compound known for its antiseptic, antioxidant, and anti-inflammatory properties. Although there is no direct evidence of 4HR's use in dental pulp regeneration, its antimicrobial and anti-inflammatory properties could be beneficial in dental procedures. 4HR has shown potential antiviral activity against respiratory viruses and SARS-CoV-2 in vitro, but further research is needed to determine its safety, efficacy, and optimal dosages for various viral infections. In the context of osteoporosis, a study found that 4HR effectively inhibited osteoclastogenesis and mitigated bone loss in an ovariectomized mouse model, suggesting that it could be a promising therapeutic option for osteoporosis. However, more research, including long-term studies, clinical trials, and comparative evaluations, is required to validate these findings and better understand 4HR's potential as a therapeutic agent in different medical applications.

Keywords 4-hexylresorcinol (4HR) · Neurologic disease · Dental pulp regeneration · Viral disease · Osteoporosis · Osteoclastogenesis

4-Hexylresorcinol (4HR) is a multifaceted compound known to interact with a variety of proteins and enzymes. The wide spectrum of biological activities it exhibits can be ascribed to its capacity to engage with multiple targets. 4HR has demonstrated antimicrobial properties, which might be due to its interaction with specific bacterial enzymes, resulting in the inhibition of bacterial growth [1]. Additionally, 4HR possesses antioxidant properties that may involve either scavenging reactive oxygen species (ROS) or inhibiting enzymes responsible for ROS generation [2]. Furthermore, 4HR has the potential to interact with certain ion channels or receptors, modulating their activity and contributing to its antinociceptive (pain-relieving) [3] or anti-inflammatory effects [4]. 4HR also can interact with specific proteins involved in protein folding or stability [5, 6]. Given this observation, 4HR could be considered a pharmacologic chaperone [7].

S.-G. Kim, *Biomedical Application of 4-Hexylresorcinol*,
https://doi.org/10.1007/978-981-97-0637-2_9

The promiscuity of 4HR in targeting multiple proteins can be both an advantage and a disadvantage. On the one hand, it may allow 4HR to exert a broad range of therapeutic effects. On the other hand, off-target interactions may lead to unintended side effects or reduced specificity in its action. It is crucial to thoroughly investigate the potential targets of 4HR and understand its mechanisms of action to harness its therapeutic potential effectively and safely.

9.1 Administration Route

4HR is indeed known to have relatively low oral bioavailability when administered per os. In a human study involving two men who received an oral dosage of 1 g of 4HR, it was observed that 18% of the dose was recovered in urine within the first 12 h, and 64% was found in fecal excretion [8]. This implies that up to 36% of the oral dosage might have been absorbed.

The dog study revealed that the absorption of 4HR varied depending on the dose and formulation. When dogs were administered a 1 g crystalline compound, 29% of the dose was detected in urine, and 67% was detected in feces, suggesting that up to 33% of the oral dosage might have been absorbed [8]. When the dose was increased to 3 g, 17% was excreted in urine, and 73% was excreted in feces, with up to 27% of the oral dosage potentially being absorbed [8].

When 4HR was administered in olive oil at a dose of 1 g, 17% of the dose was excreted in urine, and 76% was excreted in feces, indicating that up to 24% of the oral dosage might have been absorbed [8]. When the dose was increased to 3 g in olive oil, 10% was excreted in urine, and 80% was excreted in feces, suggesting that up to 20% of the oral dosage might have been absorbed [8].

This could be due to factors such as its physicochemical properties, first-pass metabolism, or poor absorption through the gastrointestinal tract [9]. Oral bioavailability refers to the percentage of an administered drug that reaches systemic circulation intact, without being broken down or metabolized in the process [9]. Low oral bioavailability can be a significant hurdle for drug development since it reduces the drug's effectiveness and may require higher doses to achieve a therapeutic effect. However, there are strategies to improve the oral bioavailability of compounds like 4HR (Fig. 9.1). A prodrug is a biologically inactive compound that is converted to the active drug inside the body. By designing a prodrug of 4HR, it might be possible to improve its absorption and bioavailability. Various drug delivery systems and formulations can be used to enhance the absorption of poorly soluble or permeable drugs, such as liposomes, nanoparticles, or solid dispersions [10]. Some compounds can enhance the absorption of drugs by altering the gastrointestinal environment or modulating the activity of transporters and enzymes [11]. Co-administering 4HR with an absorption enhancer could potentially improve its oral bioavailability.

If oral administration proves to be inefficient, alternative routes of administration, such as intravenous, intramuscular, or transdermal, could be explored to bypass the gastrointestinal absorption barriers and improve bioavailability. It is essential to

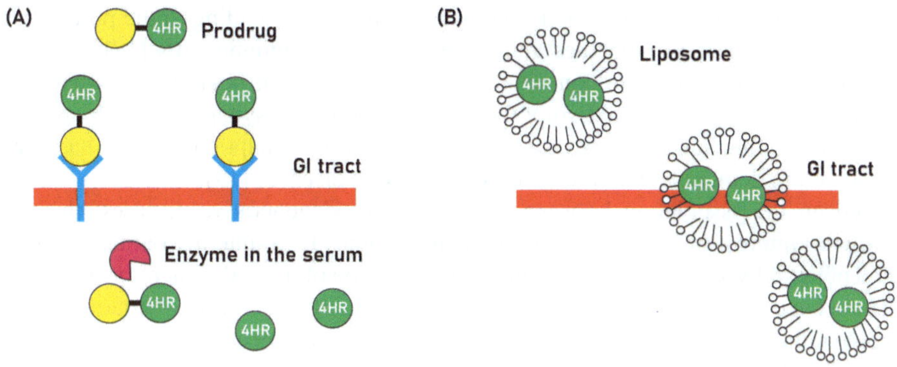

Fig. 9.1 The various approaches that can be employed to enhance the oral bioavailability of 4HR. The first strategy, as shown in (**a**), involves prodrug design. Here, a yellow circle represents a compound that enhances the absorption of 4HR from the gastrointestinal tract. Once introduced into the bloodstream, the enzyme in the serum cleaves the link between the compound and 4HR, thus enabling the latter to exert its therapeutic effects. The second strategy, as shown in (**b**), involves using liposomes as a drug delivery system. Liposomes are spherical structures composed of a lipid bilayer that can encapsulate hydrophobic compounds like 4HR. This approach allows for the targeted delivery of 4HR to the site of action, thus increasing its bioavailability and reducing the potential for side effects

keep in mind that any strategy to improve the oral bioavailability of 4HR should be carefully evaluated for safety and effectiveness before being considered for clinical use.

9.2 The Application of Neurologic Disease

Oxidative stress has been implicated in the pathogenesis of several neurodegenerative diseases, including Alzheimer's disease (AD), Parkinson's disease (PD), and other forms of dementia [12, 13]. The link between ROS and neurodegenerative disease is thought to occur through several mechanisms. Excessive ROS can cause damage to cellular components, such as proteins, lipids, and DNA, which may result in the dysfunction and death of neurons. Neuronal loss is a common feature of many neurodegenerative diseases.

Oxidative stress can lead to the misfolding and aggregation of proteins, such as amyloid-beta and tau, which are implicated in the development of Alzheimer's disease [14]. These aggregated proteins can disrupt cellular function and contribute to neuronal death. Mitochondria are the primary source of ROS, and excessive ROS production can damage mitochondrial components and impair their function [15]. Mitochondrial dysfunction has been observed in various neurodegenerative diseases and can lead to neuronal dysfunction and death [16].

ROS can activate inflammatory pathways in the brain, leading to the production of pro-inflammatory molecules and the activation of immune cells [17]. Chronic inflammation is thought to contribute to the progression of neurodegenerative diseases. Oxidative stress can disrupt the normal function of synapses, which are crucial for learning and memory processes [18]. Impaired synaptic plasticity has been observed in dementia and other neurodegenerative diseases [19].

Given the association between ROS and neurodegenerative diseases, there is growing interest in developing antioxidant therapies to counteract oxidative stress and potentially slow down or prevent the progression of neurodegenerative diseases. There have been several clinical trials investigating the use of antioxidants for the prevention or treatment of neurodegenerative diseases, such as AD and PD [20, 21]. These trials have focused on various antioxidants, including vitamins, polyphenols, and other compounds.

Several studies have investigated the potential benefits of vitamin E in AD and PD [22, 23]. Some trials showed modest benefits in slowing cognitive decline in AD patients or delaying the need for levodopa treatment in PD patients [22, 23]. However, other studies found no significant effects, and there is no clear consensus on the effectiveness of vitamin E for these conditions [24, 25]. Vitamin C has been studied for its potential neuroprotective effects, but clinical trials have not provided clear evidence for its efficacy in preventing or treating neurodegenerative diseases [23]. Further research is needed to determine if vitamin C supplementation could be beneficial in specific patient populations or at certain disease stages.

Coenzyme Q10 (CoQ10), a naturally occurring antioxidant and component of the mitochondrial electron transport chain, has been studied in several clinical trials for PD [26, 27]. The results have been mixed, with some trials showing potential benefits and others finding no significant effects. More research is needed to determine the optimal dosage, duration, and patient population for CoQ10 treatment in PD. Polyphenolic compounds, such as resveratrol and curcumin, have shown antioxidant and anti-inflammatory properties in preclinical studies, but clinical trials in neurodegenerative diseases have been limited and have not demonstrated consistent benefits [28, 29].

Although 4HR has shown various biological activities, such as antimicrobial, antioxidant, and anti-inflammatory properties, there is currently no direct evidence supporting its use as a treatment for PD or AD. To determine if 4HR could be a potential treatment for these neurodegenerative diseases, several aspects would need to be investigated:

1. Mechanism of action: It is crucial to understand the molecular targets and mechanisms through which 4HR may exert neuroprotective effects. This could involve studying its impact on protein aggregation, oxidative stress, inflammation, or other processes implicated in the pathogenesis of PD and AD.
2. Efficacy in preclinical models: Before conducting clinical trials, the efficacy of 4HR should be evaluated in preclinical models of PD and AD, such as cell cultures and animal models. This would help to determine if 4HR can provide thera-

peutic benefits in these disease contexts and inform the design of future clinical trials.

3. Pharmacokinetics and bioavailability: As previously mentioned, 4HR has low oral bioavailability. If it is to be used as a treatment for PD or AD, it may be necessary to improve its bioavailability or explore alternative routes of administration, such as intravenous, intramuscular, or transdermal delivery.
4. Safety and tolerability: Any potential treatment for PD or AD must be safe and well-tolerated by patients. Preclinical studies and clinical trials should assess the safety profile of 4HR, including any potential side effects, drug interactions, and optimal dosing regimens.

If future research demonstrates that 4HR has promising neuroprotective effects in preclinical models and a favorable safety profile, it could be considered for clinical trials in PD or AD patients. However, it is important to note that developing a new treatment for neurodegenerative diseases is a complex and lengthy process, and many potential therapies fail to demonstrate efficacy in clinical trials despite showing promise in preclinical studies.

9.3 The Application of Pulp Regeneration

Dental pulp regeneration is a promising approach in regenerative endodontics that aims to restore the vitality and function of damaged or necrotic dental pulp tissue [30]. Matrix proteins play a crucial role in this process by providing a scaffold for cell attachment, proliferation, and differentiation, as well as guiding tissue repair and regeneration [31].

Some of the matrix proteins studied for dental pulp regeneration. Dentin matrix proteins (DMPs) are critical components of the dentin extracellular matrix and play a vital role in tooth development and regeneration [32]. DMP-1 and dentin sialophospho-protein are examples of DMPs that have been investigated for their potential in dental pulp regeneration [33, 34]. These proteins have shown to promote dental pulp cell proliferation, migration, and differentiation into odontoblast-like cells, which are essential for dentin formation.

Growth factors such as bone morphogenetic proteins (BMPs), FGFs fibroblast growth factors (FGFs), and transforming growth factor-beta (TGF-β) are important regulators of cell behavior during tissue repair and regeneration. They have been studied in the context of dental pulp regeneration for their potential to stimulate dental pulp cell proliferation, migration, and differentiation, as well as promoting the formation of dentin-like structures [35, 36].

Proteins such as collagen, fibronectin, and laminin, which are major components of the extracellular matrix, have been investigated for their potential to support dental pulp regeneration [37]. These proteins can provide a scaffold for cell attachment and migration and can modulate cellular behavior during the regenerative process.

There is currently no direct evidence suggesting that 4HR could be used for dental pulp regeneration. However, given its known biological activities, it is possible that 4HR could have some potential benefits in the context of dental pulp regeneration or other aspects of dental treatment (Fig. 9.2).

4HR has demonstrated antimicrobial properties against a variety of microorganisms [1]. It could potentially be used as an adjunct in root canal treatment or other dental procedures to reduce bacterial contamination and promote better healing outcomes. 4HR's antioxidant [2, 3] and anti-inflammatory properties [4] may be beneficial in reducing inflammation and promoting tissue healing in dental procedures, although its direct impact on dental pulp regeneration remains unknown.

BMPs are a group of growth factors that belong to the TGF-β superfamily [38]. They play essential roles in various biological processes, including cell proliferation, differentiation, and tissue regeneration. In the context of dental pulp regeneration, BMPs have been shown to stimulate the differentiation of dental pulp stem cells into odontoblast-like cells, which are responsible for dentin formation [39].

According to the previous study, 4HR administration promoted the expression of bone morphogenetic protein 2 (BMP2) in primary cultured dental pulp cells [40], which is crucial for dental pulp regeneration. BMP2 is a member of the bone morphogenetic protein family, known for its roles in cell proliferation, differentiation, and tissue regeneration [38]. In the context of dental pulp regeneration, increased BMP2 expression could potentially stimulate dental pulp stem cells to differentiate into odontoblast-like cells, which are responsible for dentin formation.

Given these findings, it appears that 4HR may have potential in promoting dental pulp regeneration by increasing BMP2 expression in dental pulp cells. However, it

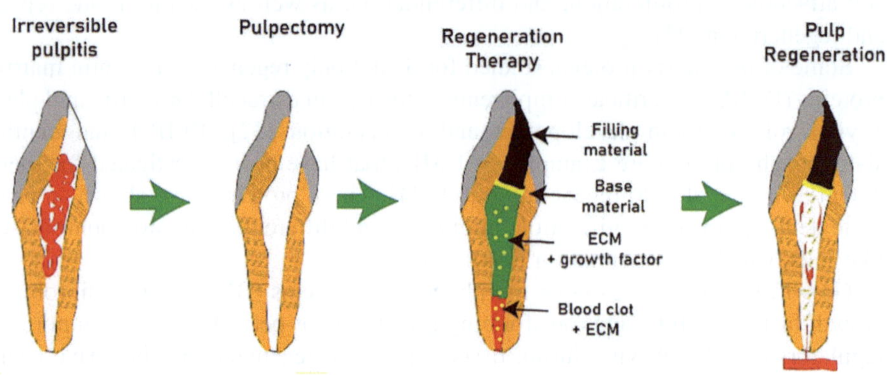

Fig. 9.2 The legend for the figure outlines the procedure for pulp regeneration. In cases of irreversible pulpitis, the inflamed pulp tissue must be removed through a process known as pulpectomy. Once this is completed, the root apex can be filed with an endodontic instrument to introduce blood originated cells into the pulp chamber. Next, the pulp chamber is filled with an extracellular matrix (ECM) that contains growth factors. This facilitates the incorporation of blood-originated cells into the ECM, which work in tandem with the growth factors to regenerate the pulp tissue. However, the use of growth factors in this procedure can be replaced by 4HR due to its ability to increase the expression level of vascular endothelial growth factor and BMPs. As a result, 4HR can facilitate the regeneration of pulp tissue without the need for external growth factors

is important to note that developing new treatment approaches is a complex and lengthy process, and many potential therapies fail to demonstrate efficacy in clinical trials despite showing promise in preclinical studies.

Clinical trials and studies using matrix proteins for dental pulp regeneration have shown promising results, with the potential to improve the outcomes of regenerative endodontic procedures. However, further research is needed to optimize the use of matrix proteins, determine the most effective combinations of proteins and growth factors, and establish standardized protocols for their application in clinical practice.

9.4 The Application for Viral Disease

Some studies have explored its potential antiviral activity against respiratory viruses, such as parainfluenza type 3 and cytomegalovirus (CMV) [41]. The study found that lozenges containing 4HR showed significant virucidal activity against both parainfluenza type 3 and CMV [41]. The authors concluded that the observed virucidal action of the 4HR-containing lozenges could contribute to the symptomatic relief of sore throat by reducing the viral load in the oropharyngeal cavity [41]. These findings suggest that 4HR may exhibit antiviral activity against certain respiratory viruses, at least in vitro. However, it is important to note that the study focuses on the virucidal activity of the lozenges rather than the direct antiviral properties of 4HR as a stand-alone compound. Furthermore, more research is needed to investigate the potential of 4HR as an antiviral agent, especially in vivo studies, and clinical trials, to determine its safety, efficacy, and optimal dosages for various viral infections.

In the study of coronavirus disease 2019 (COVID-19), the authors identified several FDA-approved drugs, including 4HR, that showed potential antiviral activity against SARS-CoV-2 in vitro [42]. Specifically, they found that 4HR demonstrated antiviral activity at nontoxic concentrations in Vero E6 cells [42]. Additionally, they reported that 4HR might target the host enzyme PLA2G16, which plays a role in the life cycle of SARS-CoV-2 [42]. These findings suggest that 4HR may have potential antiviral activity against SARS-CoV-2 in vitro, and it could be a candidate for further investigation as a repurposable drug for treating COVID-19. However, it is important to note that these results are based on in vitro studies, and more research is needed, including in vivo studies and clinical trials, to evaluate the safety, efficacy, and optimal dosages of 4HR for use as an antiviral treatment for SARS-CoV-2 infection.

4HR has been shown to bind to DNA and stabilize its structure [43]. DNA bound to 4HR exhibits increased resistance to ultraviolet radiation [44]. Given the structural similarity between DNA and RNA, it is plausible that 4HR could also bind to RNA. This binding may result in the stabilization of DNA or RNA, potentially leading to replication resistance. If 4HR binds to viral DNA or RNA, the stabilization may render the genetic material non-replicable. Consequently, this could be beneficial in controlling viral diseases by inhibiting viral replication.

9.5 The Application for Osteoporosis

Osteoporosis is a widespread condition affecting both genders, but it is more common in women, especially postmenopausal women [45]. This disease involves a reduction in bone density, resulting in fragile bones and a heightened risk of fractures [46]. Millions of people globally suffer from osteoporosis, with elderly women facing higher risks due to hormonal changes during menopause [45].

Several factors account for the increased prevalence of osteoporosis in women, including their generally lower bone mass compared to men, which heightens their risk of bone loss [45, 47]. Estrogen, a hormone crucial for bone health, decreases significantly during menopause, causing rapid bone mass loss [47]. Additionally, women generally outlive men, meaning they may experience more postmenopausal years during which bone loss can occur.

Osteoporosis can lead to severe complications, primarily due to the weakened bone structure and elevated fracture risk [45]. Fractures in the hip, spine, and wrist become more likely, which can result in chronic pain, disability, and loss of independence. Hip fractures are particularly concerning, as they often necessitate surgery and can cause extended immobility, potentially leading to further complications [48]. Osteoporosis can also cause vertebral compression fractures, leading to intense back pain, height loss, and spinal deformities such as kyphosis (hunched-forward posture) or scoliosis (abnormal spinal curvature) [49]. These spinal deformities can reduce lung space, impairing lung function and increasing the risk of respiratory problems like pneumonia.

Various medications are available to prevent and treat osteoporosis-related complications, but they can also have side effects or adverse effects. It's crucial to balance the medication's potential benefits against the risks of side effects. Common osteoporosis medications can have possible adverse effects, such as gastrointestinal issues, atypical femur fractures, and osteonecrosis of the jaw from bisphosphonates [50]; hot flashes, leg cramps, and a slightly increased risk of blood clots and stroke from selective estrogen receptor modulators [51]; leg cramps, dizziness, nausea, and a low risk of osteosarcoma (a rare bone cancer) from parathyroid hormone-related protein analogs and recombinant human parathyroid hormone [52, 53]; low calcium levels, skin infections, and osteonecrosis of the jaw in rare cases from denosumab [54]; and nasal irritation, gastrointestinal issues, and an increased risk of certain cancers with long-term use from calcitonin [55, 56].

A previous study explored 4HR, a small organic compound known for its antiseptic and antioxidant properties, and its role in osteoclastogenesis [57]. Mouse-derived bone marrow macrophages were used to study 4HR's effects on osteogenesis, while an ovariectomy (OVX) mouse model was used to examine its in vivo effects, with histological analysis. The results indicated that 4HR effectively inhibited osteoclastogenesis induced by receptor activator of NF-κB ligand (RANKL) in a dose-dependent manner [57]. Additionally, 4HR substantially reduced osteoclast-specific markers expression and inhibited osteoclastogenesis by blocking the activation of the NF-κB signaling pathway [57]. Consistent with in vitro findings, 4HR mitigated OVX-induced bone loss and considerably decreased the osteoclast count in the proximal tibia in vivo [57]. These results suggest that 4HR could be a promising new therapeutic option for osteoporosis.

However, the study had some limitations, including the use of an ovariectomized mouse model, which may not fully represent human biological processes. The translation of these results to human populations should be done with caution. The study focused on the effects of 4HR on osteoclastogenesis and bone loss, and it would be helpful to compare the efficacy and safety of 4HR with other currently available osteoporosis treatments to better understand its potential advantages and disadvantages. The study may not have investigated the long-term effects of 4HR on bone loss and osteoporosis management. Further research is needed to evaluate the safety and efficacy of 4HR over an extended period.

To address these limitations, future studies should consider conducting long-term investigations, exploring potential side effects, and comparing the effects of 4HR with existing treatments. Additionally, conducting clinical trials in human populations would help to validate the results from this animal study and provide a better understanding of 4HR's potential as a therapeutic agent for osteoporosis.

9.6 Closing Remarks

4HR has been utilized in a variety of industries such as antiseptic, food, and cosmetics. This compound has demonstrated efficacy as an antiseptic due to its ability to inhibit the growth of microorganisms. In the food industry, it is commonly used as a preservative due to its ability to prevent discoloration and spoilage in certain products. Additionally, 4HR is frequently employed within cosmetics due to its antioxidant and skin-whitening properties.

This book explores the potential applications of 4HR in various fields, drawing upon relevant literature to provide insight into its potential uses. This chapter dedicated to the limitations and unexplored areas of 4HR usage aims to identify any potential drawbacks or areas where further research is required. It is important to understand the limitations of any compound to ensure its safe and effective use.

While this book provides a comprehensive overview of 4HR applications, it is important to note that certain areas have not been explored in detail. There may be additional industries or applications where 4HR can prove useful that are not covered within the scope of this book. Therefore, further research and exploration may be necessary to fully understand the potential of 4HR in various fields.

References

1. Matthews D, Adegoke O, Shephard A (2020) Bactericidal activity of hexylresorcinol lozenges against oropharyngeal organisms associated with acute sore throat. BMC Res Notes 13:99
2. Yen GC, Duh PD, Lin CW (2003) Effects of resveratrol and 4-hexylresorcinol on hydrogen peroxide-induced oxidative DNA damage in human lymphocytes. Free Radic Res 37(5):509–514

3. Brizzi A, Aiello F, Boccella S et al (2020) Synthetic bioactive olivetol-related amides: the influence of the phenolic group in cannabinoid receptor activity. Bioorg Med Chem 28(11):115513
4. Kim YS, Kim DW, Kim SG, Lee SK (2020) 4-hexylresorcinol-induced protein expression changes in human umbilical cord vein endothelial cells as determined by immunoprecipitation high-performance liquid chromatography. PLoS One 15(12):e0243975
5. Lee JH, Kweon H, Oh JH et al (2022) 4-hexylresorcinol treatment before degumming increases the β-sheet structure of silk Sericin and BMP-2 expression in RAW264.7 cells. Int J Mol Sci 24(1):150
6. Kang YJ, Yang WG, Chae WS, Kim DW, Kim SG, Rotaru H (2022) Administration of 4-hexylresorcinol increases p53-mediated transcriptional activity in oral cancer cells with the p53 mutation. Oncol Rep 48(3):160
7. Kim SG (2022) 4-hexylresorcinol: pharmacologic chaperone and its application for wound healing. Maxillofac Plast Reconstr Surg 44:5
8. WHO Food Additive Series 35 (2005) 4-Hexylresorcinol (136–77-6). https://www.inchem.org/documents/jecfa/jecmono/v35je04.htm
9. Dahan A, Beig A, Lindley D, Miller JM (2016) The solubility-permeability interplay and oral drug formulation design: two heads are better than one. Adv Drug Deliv Rev 101:99–107
10. Savjani KT, Gajjar AK, Savjani JK (2012) Drug solubility: importance and enhancement techniques. ISRN Pharm 2012:195727
11. Aungst BJ (2000) Intestinal permeation enhancers. J Pharm Sci 89(4):429–442
12. Butterfield DA, Halliwell B (2019) Oxidative stress, dysfunctional glucose metabolism and Alzheimer disease. Nat Rev Neurosci 20(3):148–160
13. Dias V, Junn E, Mouradian MM (2013) The role of oxidative stress in Parkinson's disease. J Parkinsons Dis 3(4):461–491
14. Butterfield DA, Swomley AM, Sultana R (2013) Amyloid β-peptide (1-42)-induced oxidative stress in Alzheimer disease: importance in disease pathogenesis and progression. Antioxid Redox Signal 19(8):823–835
15. Murphy MP (2009) How mitochondria produce reactive oxygen species. Biochem J 417(1):1–13
16. Lin MT, Beal MF (2006) Mitochondrial dysfunction and oxidative stress in neurodegenerative diseases. Nature 443(7113):787–795
17. Glass CK, Saijo K, Winner B, Marchetto MC, Gage FH (2010) Mechanisms underlying inflammation in neurodegeneration. Cell 140(6):918–934
18. Serrano F, Klann E (2004) Reactive oxygen species and synaptic plasticity in the aging hippocampus. Ageing Res Rev 3(4):431–443
19. Citri A, Malenka RC (2008) Synaptic plasticity: multiple forms, functions, and mechanisms. Neuropsychopharmacology 33(1):18–41
20. Galasko DR, Peskind E, Clark CM et al (2012) Antioxidants for Alzheimer disease: a randomized clinical trial with cerebrospinal fluid biomarker measures. Arch Neurol 69(7):836–841
21. Beal MF (2003) Bioenergetic approaches for neuroprotection in Parkinson's disease. Ann Neurol 53(Suppl 3):S39–S47
22. Sano M, Ernesto C, Thomas RG et al (1997) A controlled trial of selegiline, alpha-tocopherol, or both as treatment for Alzheimer's disease. The Alzheimer's disease cooperative study. N Engl J Med 336(17):1216–1222
23. Fahn S (1992) A pilot trial of high-dose alpha-tocopherol and ascorbate in early Parkinson's disease. Ann Neurol 32(Suppl):S128–S132
24. Dysken MW, Sano M, Asthana S et al (2014) Effect of vitamin E and memantine on functional decline in Alzheimer disease: the TEAM-AD VA cooperative randomized trial. JAMA 311(1):33–44
25. Parkinson Study Group (1993) Effects of tocopherol and deprenyl on the progression of disability in early Parkinson's disease. N Engl J Med 328(3):176–183
26. Beal MF, Oakes D, Shoulson I et al (2014) A randomized clinical trial of high-dosage coenzyme Q10 in early Parkinson disease: no evidence of benefit. JAMA Neurol 71(5):543–552

27. Shults CW, Oakes D, Kieburtz K et al (2002) Effects of coenzyme Q10 in early Parkinson disease: evidence of slowing of the functional decline. Arch Neurol 59(10):1541–1550
28. Turner RS, Thomas RG, Craft S et al (2015) A randomized, double-blind, placebo-controlled trial of resveratrol for Alzheimer disease. Neurology 85(16):1383–1391
29. Ringman JM, Frautschy SA, Teng E et al (2012) Oral curcumin for Alzheimer's disease: tolerability and efficacy in a 24-week randomized, double blind, placebo-controlled study. Alzheimers Res Ther 4(5):43
30. Mao JJ, Kim SG, Zhou J et al (2012) Regenerative endodontics: barriers and strategies for clinical translation. Dent Clin N Am 56:639–649
31. Minic S, Vital S, Chaussain C, Boukpessi T, Mangione F (2022) Tissue characteristics in endodontic regeneration: a systematic review. Int J Mol Sci 23(18):10534
32. Ravindran S, George A (2014) Multifunctional ECM proteins in bone and teeth. Exp Cell Res 325(2):148–154
33. Machla F, Sokolova V, Platania V et al (2023) Tissue engineering at the dentin-pulp interface using human treated dentin scaffolds conditioned with DMP1 or BMP2 plasmid DNA-carrying calcium phosphate nanoparticles. Acta Biomater 159:156–172
34. Kim D, Lee H, Lee GH, Hoang TH, Kim HR, Kim GH (2022) Fabrication of bone-derived decellularized extracellular matrix/ceramic-based biocomposites and their osteo/odontogenic differentiation ability for dentin regeneration. Bioeng Transl Med 7(3):e10317
35. Ishimatsu H, Kitamura C, Morotomi T et al (2009) Formation of dentinal bridge on surface of regenerated dental pulp in dentin defects by controlled release of fibroblast growth factor-2 from gelatin hydrogels. J Endod 35(6):858–865
36. Zhang W, Yelick PC (2010) Vital pulp therapy-current progress of dental pulp regeneration and revascularization. Int J Dent 2010:856087
37. Galler KM, D'Souza RN, Hartgerink JD (2010) Biomaterials and their potential applications for dental tissue engineering. J Mater Chem 20(40):8730–8746
38. Wu M, Chen G, Li YP (2016) TGF-β and BMP signaling in osteoblast, skeletal development, and bone formation, homeostasis and disease. Bone Res 4:16009
39. Nakashima M (2005) Bone morphogenetic proteins in dentin regeneration for potential use in endodontic therapy. Cytokine Growth Factor Rev 16(3):369–376
40. Kim JH, Kim DW, Kim SG, Kim TW (2020) 4-hexylresorcinol administration increases dental hard tissue formation and incisor eruption rate in rats. Appl Sci 10(16):5511
41. Shephard A, Zybeshari S (2015) Virucidal action of sore throat lozenges against respiratory viruses parainfluenza type 3 and cytomegalovirus. Antivir Res 123:158–162
42. Chen F, Shi Q, Pei F et al (2021) A systems-level study reveals host-targeted repurposable drugs against SARS-CoV-2 infection. Mol Syst Biol 17(8):e10239
43. Davydova OK, Deriabin DG, Nikiian AN, El'-Registan GI (2005) Mechanisms of interaction between DNA and chemical analogues of microbial anabiosis autoinducers. Mikrobiologiia 74(5):616–625
44. Davydova OK, Deriabin DG, El'-Registan GI (2006) Influence of chemical analogues of microbial autoregulators on the sensitivity of DNA to UV radiation. Mikrobiologiia 75(5):654–661
45. Salari N, Darvishi N, Bartina Y et al (2021) Global prevalence of osteoporosis among the world older adults: a comprehensive systematic review and meta-analysis. J Orthop Surg Res 16(1):669
46. Coughlan T, Dockery F (2014) Osteoporosis and fracture risk in older people. Clin Med (Lond) 14(2):187–191
47. De Martinis M, Sirufo MM, Polsinelli M, Placidi G, Di Silvestre D, Ginaldi L (2021) Gender differences in osteoporosis: a single-center observational study. World J Mens Health 39(4):750–759
48. Fuggle NR, Curtis EM, Ward KA, Harvey NC, Dennison EM, Cooper C (2019) Fracture prediction, imaging and screening in osteoporosis. Nat Rev Endocrinol 15(9):535–547
49. Kutsal FY, Ergin Ergani GO (2021) Vertebral compression fractures: still an unpredictable aspect of osteoporosis. Turk J Med Sci 51(2):393–399

50. Reyes C, Hitz M, Prieto-Alhambra D, Abrahamsen B (2016) Risks and benefits of bisphosphonate therapies. J Cell Biochem 117(1):20–28
51. Farkas S, Szabó A, Hegyi AE et al (2022) Estradiol and estrogen-like alternative therapies in use: the importance of the selective and non-classical actions. Biomedicines 10(4):861
52. Uihlein AV, Leder BZ (2012) Anabolic therapies for osteoporosis. Endocrinol Metab Clin N Am 41(3):507–525
53. Subbiah V, Madsen VS, Raymond AK, Benjamin RS, Ludwig JA (2010) Of mice and men: divergent risks of teriparatide-induced osteosarcoma. Osteoporos Int 21(6):1041–1045
54. Goulden EL, Crowley RK (2023) When and how to stop denosumab therapy in a patient with osteoporosis. Clin Endocrinol 98(5):649–653
55. Knopp JA, Diner BM, Blitz M, Lyritis GP, Rowe BH (2005) Calcitonin for treating acute pain of osteoporotic vertebral compression fractures: a systematic review of randomized, controlled trials. Osteoporos Int 16(10):1281–1290
56. Wells G, Chernoff J, Gilligan JP, Krause DS (2016) Does salmon calcitonin cause cancer? A review and meta-analysis. Osteoporos Int 27(1):13–19
57. Yi W, Liu T, Gao X, Xie Y, Liu M (2021) 4-hexylresorcinol inhibits osteoclastogenesis by suppressing the NF-κB signaling pathway and reverses bone loss in ovariectomized mice. Exp Ther Med 21(4):354

MIX
Papier aus verantwortungsvollen Quellen
Paper from responsible sources
FSC® C105338

If you have any concerns about our products,
you can contact us on
ProductSafety@springernature.com

In case Publisher is established outside the EU,
the EU authorized representative is:
Springer Nature Customer Service Center GmbH
Europaplatz 3, 69115 Heidelberg, Germany

Printed by Libri Plureos GmbH
in Hamburg, Germany